TENNISBPM

TENNIS FITNESS

(TENNIS BODY PERFORMANCE MATRIX)
LOSE FAT, EAT BETTER,
PERFORM MORE, PREVENT INJURY,
AND REST SMART
(FOR KIDS, TEENS, ADULTS, TRAINERS & COACHES)

RANIL HARSHANA

ISBN: 1492867969
ISBN 13: 9781492867968
Library of Congress Control Number: 2013919137
CreateSpace Independent Publishing Platform
North Charleston, South Carolina

To Juan Carlos Santana MD, CSCS
For inspiring, motivating, and educating me. You have helped enhance my personal and professional life by being a great mentor and a friend.

ACKNOWLEDGMENTS

I would like to thank Suresh Menon for providing me with the opportunity to share my fitness knowledge and experience with the worldwide tennis community and also for mentoring me for presentations and workshops.

A thank you to Miguel Crespo, PhD, for providing me with the opportunity to share my knowledge with tennis coaches and for helping me in the preparation of this manual and finding answers to tennis-related queries.

I would also thank the following individuals for appearing in the photographs and participating in Tennis BPM. Most of all, thank you for being awesome students, athletes, and friends over the years.

1. Nadine Jayaratne
2. Joshua Jayaratne
3. Dhanya Madugalle
4. Zehra Ozdemir

I am grateful to Manisha and Lashan Wanigatunga, who helped organize the book content, website design, and marketing and Kasun Malinda for the photographs.

It was an honor to work with all of you tennis coaches. I appreciate the learning experience I acquired training tennis players for international tournaments with Dominquez Utzigner, Juan Nunez, Aad Zawan, Philip Su, Jagath Welikala, and Upul Priyantha and their invaluable tips and guidance in training my tennis athletes to an international level of competition.

CONTENTS

Introduction 1
  Why Play Tennis? 2
    Common Reasons to Play Tennis 2
  Benefits of Tennis BPM 5
  Pre–Tennis Participation Questionnaire (PTPQ) 6
  Components of Tennis Fitness 8
    How Your Body Utilizes Energy for Movement 9
Section 1—Warm-Up 10
Section 2—Cardiovascular Fitness for Tennis 17
  Benefits of Training with This System 17
  Aerobic Capacity (VO2 Max) 17
  Cardiovascular Exercises 18
Section 3—Stability (Balance) 21
  Body Weight Stability Training 21
  Core Stability Training 21
Section 4—Coordination 27
Section 5—Muscle Size, Strength, Endurance, and Power 31
  Benefits of Strength and Resistance Training 31
  Legs 35
  Chest 43
  Back 48
  Arms 54
  Shoulders 58
  Abdominals 63
  Lower Back 67
Section 6—Speed and Agility 71
  Speed 71
  Agility 72

Section 7—Reaction and Quickness 79
    Plyometrics 83
Section 8—Cooldown and Static Flexibility 84
    Static Stretching 84
Section 9—Nutrition 96
    Hydration 96
    Dehydration 97
    Rehydration 97
    Why Nutrition Is Key 98
    Need Food 99
    Carbohydrates 99
    What Is the Glycemic Index? (GI Index) 100
    Protein 101
    Why Protein Is Your Repair Tool 101
    Fat and Lipids 102
    Benefits of Fat 103
    Benefits of Cholesterol 104
    Vitamins 104
    Minerals 106
    Want Food 107
        Processed, Refined, and Inorganic Food 107
    How to Select Food 107
        Four Reasons to Put Something Back on the Shelf 108
        Three Reasons to Take Food Home 109
Section 10—Importance of Recovery and Rest 110
    Sleep 110
    Relaxation 112
Sample Programs for Kids, Teens, and Adults 114
Final Note 117
Warning 118
Bibliography 119

INTRODUCTION

As a fitness trainer and conditioning coach, I have trained many tennis players participating in the junior and senior Davis Cup, the Fed Cup, and even at the Paralympic Games. I have also come across and trained athletes in many other sports such as rugby, basketball, swimming, martial arts, and track. The main reason they are able to perform well and prevent injuries is because of their support team of medical professionals, physiotherapists, conditioning and performance coaches, dietitians, massage therapists and sport-specific coaches.

When compared with noncompetitive tennis players regardless of age, the number of professionals is much smaller. Considering the ages of players that range from five to over eighty years old, noncompetitive tennis could be the most sought-after sport worldwide. Most people enjoy the game of tennis for the competition, recreation, socialization, or other reasons.

The purpose behind this book is to educate the basic-level tennis coaches, personal and group fitness trainers, parents, and individuals on how to gradually progress in tennis-specific fitness and then combine it with tennis. After you read the material and apply the instructions, you will know how to prevent injury, attain your fitness goals, and improve your tennis game.

I'm certain many fitness and tennis professionals would agree with me when I say, "You have to be fit to play tennis," rather than the old saying, "Play tennis to be fit."

The final section of this book provides fitness protocols for kids, teens, and adults from my total body fitness solution, Tennis BPM (body performance matrix). Following these guidelines will help reduce health risks, burn fat, and aid with toning as well as other benefits.

Compared to other fitness methods and sports, tennis-related fitness offers a well-rounded fitness solution. Anyone can do these exercises as an individual, a group, a couple, or a family. The tools in this book will enable you to perform any activity with ease, and they include movements we use in daily life, such as sudden sprints, quick reaction, and running in different directions.

WHY PLAY TENNIS?

Let us explore a few of the common reasons why people of various age groups and genders play the wonderful game of tennis.

For the scope of this book, I will only cover the exercises appropriate for recreational players and junior players. This is not intended for junior or senior competitive players. They need the guidance and support of qualified tennis coaches, conditioning specialists, and dietitians; each of these professionals brings his or her students highly specialized skills and knowledge.

Common Reasons to Play Tennis

1) **Kids (Ages 5–12)**
   At this tender age, kids are in the initial stages of experiencing life and development. Here are a few reasons why they would start to play tennis.

   Kids' Mentality
   - I want to play because my friends and family do.
   - I saw someone play tennis on the television.
   - I want to be like my role model in tennis.
   - I like hitting the balls with the tennis racket and running around.

   Parents' Mentality
   - We would like our child to learn a sport.
   - We want him or her to move and lose weight because of a sedentary lifestyle.
   - We want the child to play competitive tennis.
   - We hope to groom our child to be a world class player.

   Things to Remember
   At this age, kids are still developing mentally and physically. They must make gradual progress without too much mental or physical strain since they are developing coordination at this age. As parents, do not let them specialize in playing a single sport. If you do, it will overexert their muscles and bones, making them injury prone.

   Children who are introduced to a variety of sports will benefit from the positive effects of overall movement, coordination, balance, speed, reaction, flexibility, and cardiovascular fitness found in basketball, touch rugby, and swimming. These are the best complementary sports at this stage, and they improve motor skills (coordinated movements of nerves, muscles, and bones).

Parents should find a tennis coach with proper credentials and look into the fitness training aspect to prevent injuries.

2) **Teens (Ages 13–18)**
Biologically, this is when hormones start to activate and reach their potential in both genders. This is also the age that kids start to experiment with life, and attitudes lead the way.

Teens' Mentality
- To impress friends
- To get a college scholarship
- For the love of the game
- As a social activity
- To get into the professional competition circuit

Parents' Mentality
With or without being forced, teens will get involved in tennis at this age. Teens may participate voluntarily, spending many hours on tennis and neglecting recovery because of other sports and activities, unhealthy eating patterns, or will attempt to become champions overnight.

<u>Things to Remember</u>
Have a discussion with your teen and help him or her set future goals. If the teen is interested in pursuing tennis as a competitive sport, discuss this with a coach and draw up a plan accordingly.

3) **Adults**
Due to a fast-paced life with work, family, friends, and many other factors, most people find it hard to find the time to be healthy and fit, especially to play a sport at this age.

Adult Mentality
- To socialize
- To lose weight or fat and shape up
- To improve overall fitness
- To play in recreational tennis tournaments

Therefore, for adults, playing tennis is mainly about getting in shape, relaxing, improving health and fitness, and reducing stress.

There are sample workout plans at the end of the book providing a total body workout with tennis-specific fitness in thirty to forty minutes.

Individual requirements for each individual and age group may differ. Carefully read all the sections in this book so that you will understand how to progress gradually.

Do not hesitate to refer to an appropriate professional when needed. A proper foundation of tennis-related fitness and technical form will enhance your performance for a weekend game of tennis or give you an energetic, calorie-burning program.

BENEFITS OF TENNIS BPM

1. Cost effective: you can do it on clay or hard courts, in parks or even at home.
2. It can be done as a family, with friends, as a couple, or individually.
3. It uses simple and affordable equipment (tennis balls and cans, basketball, medicine ball, bands, dumbbells, piece of chalk) compared to expensive memberships to gyms and fitness centers.
4. Compared with the current trends in workouts Tennis BPM has the extra advantage of:
    - Improving stability (balance)
    - Improving total body coordination
    - Improving reaction and response
    - Improving physical movement in sudden change of direction
    - Practicing acceleration and deceleration

If you make Tennis BPM a regular workout to supplement your existing exercise routines, you will see why tennis players have the best overall fitness and physique.

With the increase of sedentary lifestyles, people are experiencing various health issues. It is advisable to undergo medical and fitness evaluations before participating in tennis. This will accelerate your fitness goals and allow you to participate in tennis in an injury-free environment. Using the Tennis BPM program as part of tennis training will give kids a proper athletic foundation.

PRE–TENNIS PARTICIPATION QUESTIONNAIRE (PTPQ)

Filling out this questionnaire will help to identify your condition before you participate in tennis and fitness programs. If you answer yes to numbers nine through fifteen, please seek medical advice before pursuing physical activity. You may also want to consult a dietitian, physiotherapist, performance coach and a tennis coach.

1. Name
2. Age
3. Sex
4. Weight
5. Height
6. What other activities or sports do you participate in?
7. Amount of time per week (hours) you do the above mentioned activities:
8. Have you played tennis before?
    a. If yes, at what level (beginner, recreational, competitive)?
9. Do you have a family history of diabetes, cancer or heart disease?
10. Have you ever experienced pain in the heart or have difficulty breathing?
11. Do you suffer from headaches, dizziness or blurred vision?
12. Have you had any pain or problems in a knee, ankle, shoulder, wrist, neck, hip or any other joint or muscle?
13. Do you have any allergies (dust, pollen etc.)?
14. Do you feel any discomfort while doing any physical activity?
15. What is your blood pressure, blood sugar, and lipid profile?
16. Do you smoke?
17. What is your blood type?
18. In case of emergency, contact:
19. Are you taking any kind of medication or supplements?
20. How many days per week do you wish to participate in tennis?
21. What is your goal in participation?

Before you start to play tennis, don't forget to select the following items.

1) **Racket**

   It is very important to use a good racket with the proper weight, string tension, and grip; this will prevent undue injury and improve your playing standards. Talk with a tennis professional, ideally one certified by ITF, USTA or Tennis Australia, as these professionals are trained and familiar with good standards.

2) **Sunblock**

   If you like to play in the sun or do your fitness training on outdoor courts, it's advisable that you invest in proper sunscreen lotion with an SPF (sun protection factor) of forty to sixty.

3) **Sun-protective clothing**

   With the rapid development of sports science, you can now select from a wide variety of high-tech performance clothing depending on the climate, sport, and many other factors. Keep your eyes open for clothing with a sweat evaporation system, muscle compression capabilities, SPF, cold-weather protection etc.

4) **Shoes**

   The best pair of shoes depends on whether you will be using a hard court or a clay court. When you shop for shoes, make sure they fit and that the surface has a good cushioning system and proper gripping. You should also consider the weight of the shoes.

COMPONENTS OF TENNIS FITNESS

Tennis at a professional level is very demanding and can be rated among the toughest sports. It requires cardiovascular fitness, muscle strength, endurance, power, speed, agility, reaction, balance, tactical thinking, coordination, and concentration. On some occasions, a tennis match will last close to four hours if it is a five-set match.

However, the scope of this book is recreational tennis, where a match will typically last for two or three sets in the time span of one or two hours. If you are a fitness enthusiast, you may already spend thirty to sixty minutes on your workouts.

Whether you play tennis professionally or recreationally, tennis requires fitness at all levels. You will need to move properly and keep moving till the end of the specified number of sets.

The below skills are required at any level of tennis.

Skills (and applications) required for tennis	Corresponding daily activities
Warm up—gearing up for the task at hand	Starting your day
Cardiovascular fitness—lasting the number of sets	Sightseeing, walking in shopping malls, hiking, backpacking etc.
Power—serving	Playing with your kids, friends, or family—throwing objects like a ball
Muscle strength and endurance—rallying and court movement	Climbing stairs, playing sports like beach volleyball, soccer, football, or basketball
Speed and agility—getting to the ball fast and directional changes	Running to catch a cab, rushing on the subway platform, weekend recreational sports, running behind kids etc.
Stability (balance)—getting into a proper stance before a stroke	Stepping down stairs, balancing when walking on slippery floors or uneven surfaces
Reaction—anticipation and reacting to strokes of opponent	Trying to get out of harm's way if an object comes towards you or trying to grasp a breakable object you dropped

Tactical thinking—knowing tennis strategies and maneuvers	Planning the next move that will be beneficial in your business or personal life
Coordination—getting one's act together	Brushing your teeth, pushing a cabinet, or moving a table
Cooldown	Relaxing and going to sleep

How Your Body Utilizes Energy for Movement

1-2-3 Energy Transfers

As we breathe, eat, and move, the body converts oxygen and food into energy.

Your body functions rely on three energy systems. Each one is interdependent and gives us energy to cruise through the day, week, and year. I will try to describe this complicated physiological process in a simple manner.

Tennis is one of the few sports which require your body to use all three energy systems.

System 1: Lasts for five to ten seconds (short rallies in a tennis match, 100-meter sprint)
       Uses energy compound derived from body
       Explosive energy for high-speed activities

System 2: Lasts fifteen seconds to one or two minutes (long rallies, 400-meter and 800-meter races)
       Uses carbohydrates as energy
       Medium-speed activities

System 3: Lasts from over two minutes up to a couple of hours (tennis match, hiking, or marathon running)
       Uses oxygen for energy
       Gives energy for System 2
       Slow-speed activities

SECTION 1 — WARM-UP

To describe it in a few words, a warm-up prepares your body for the task at hand.

In fitness, it can be defined as increasing your body temperature and circulation throughout the body so that you won't get injured while playing tennis or participating in fitness training. This is a mandatory step before any activity that requires movement.

Usually, people do static stretching (holding the stretch) to warm up, but this is not recommended; this type of stretch resets the muscle back to its resting level. Static stretches are ideal to incorporate at the end of your workday or after playing tennis or other sports. Think of it as if you are preparing your body to rest.

In modern-day sports, we start with dynamic flexibility (light movement gearing up for the sports activity). Tennis-specific movement patterns are listed below, then gradually building to the speed of motion that will be used in tennis (differs from sport to sport). Descriptions for these exercises follow the overview provided here.

1) Butt kicks
2) Knee hops
3) Propeller
4) Side karate chop
5) Hamstring march (with arms)
6) Step over hurdle backward (outside to inside)
7) Step over hurdle forward (inside to outside)
8) Arm circle forward with toes up
9) Arm circle backward with toes down
10) Crossover balance lunge

Benefits
- Increases heart rate
- Increases oxygen in blood
- Increases synovial fluid and reduce friction between joints
- Develops speed of nerve impulses to communicate with muscle contractions
- Increases force and speed of muscle contractions
- Increases elasticity and extensibility of muscle fibers
- Decreases blood thickness, letting the oxygen travel to different body parts more easily

Duration: Five to Ten Minutes

Note: Each of the above exercises can be repeated twice from doubles line to doubles on one side of the court.

1) Butt Kicks

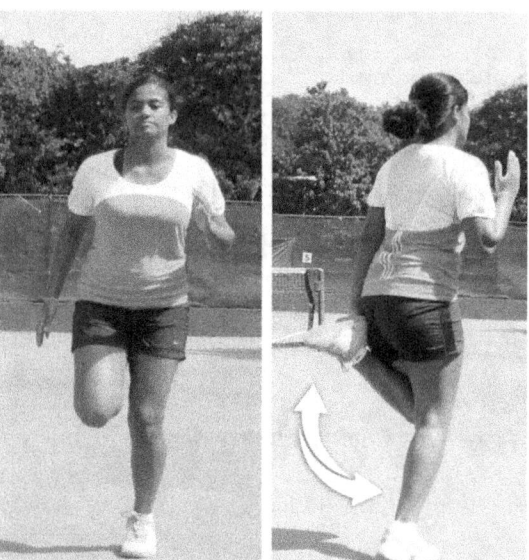

- Stand either at the doubles line to doubles or baseline to net on one side of the tennis court.
- When kicking, make sure your heels touch your buttocks as you move rhythmically.
- Always land on the balls of your feet.

2) Alternate Knee Hops

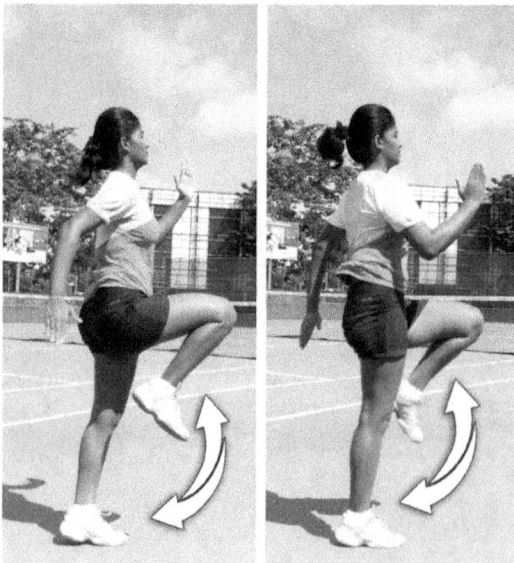

- Make sure you get a slight explosive movement when doing this exercise.
- When you hop, make sure you counter your balance with the opposite hand as shown.

3) Propeller

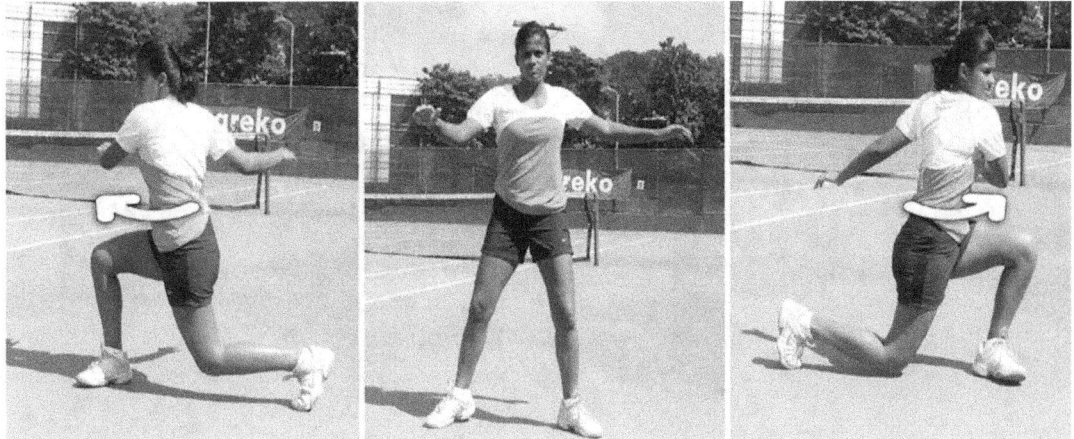

- Refer to the center photo as the starting point. Stand with feet spread shoulder-width apart and arms extended.
- From that position, rotate and lunge to right or left side as shown.
- Come back to the starting point.
- Repeat on the opposite side.

4) Side Karate Chop

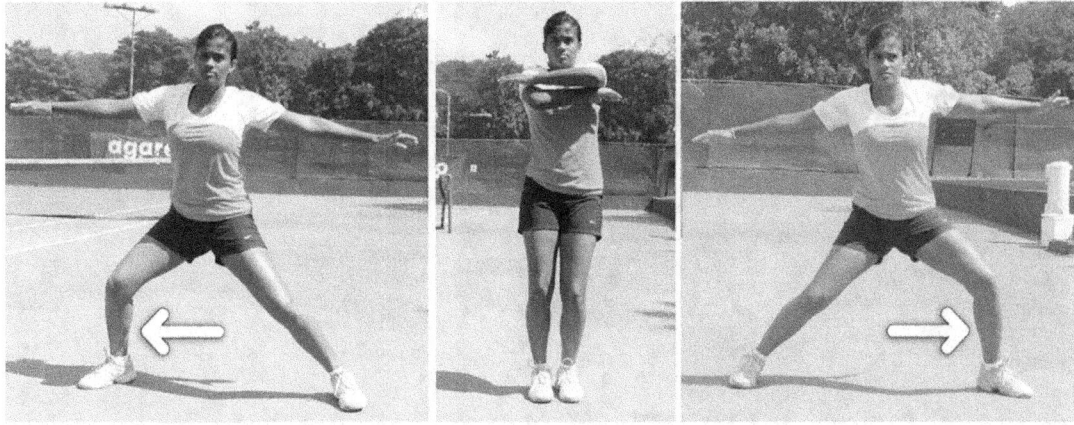

- Start with feet together, as seen on the center photo, with arms placed left over right or vice versa.
- Step to the right or left, keeping one foot stationary.
- As you step, uncross your arms and extend them.
- Return to the starting position and repeat on the other side.

5) Hamstring March

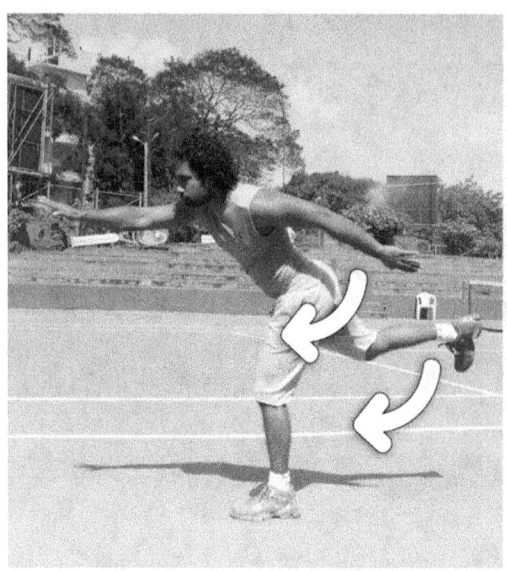 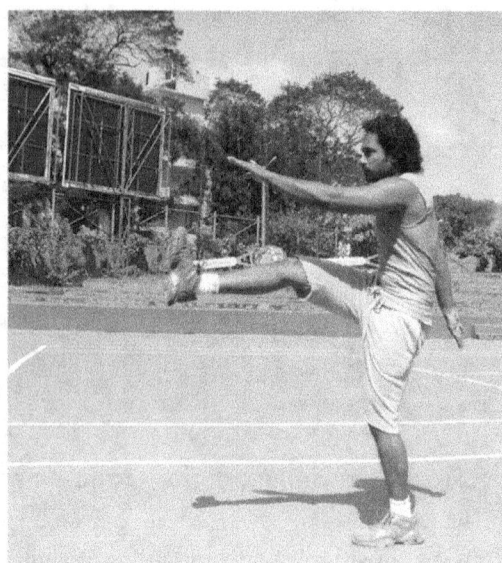

- Keeping one knee slightly bent and using slight momentum, try to swing your opposite arm and leg.
- Don't make any sudden movements.
- Gradually increase the speed and the range of the swinging motion.

6) Step Out and Over Hurdles

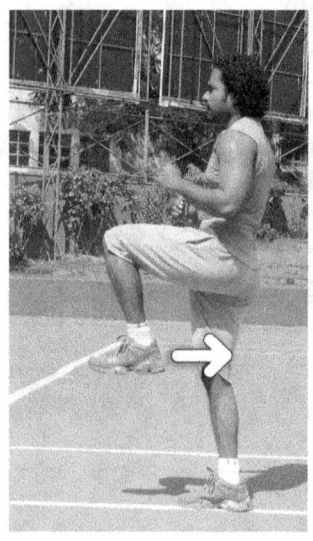 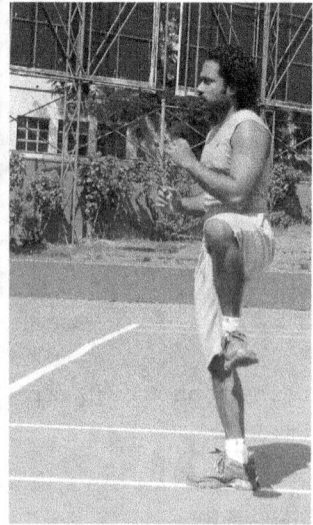

- Start with your feet together and look straight ahead.
- Lift the left leg as shown and imagine you are moving backward while stepping over hurdles.
- Repeat with right leg.

7) Step In and Over Hurdles

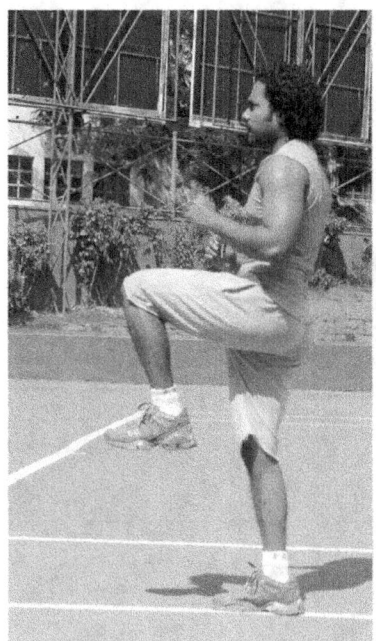 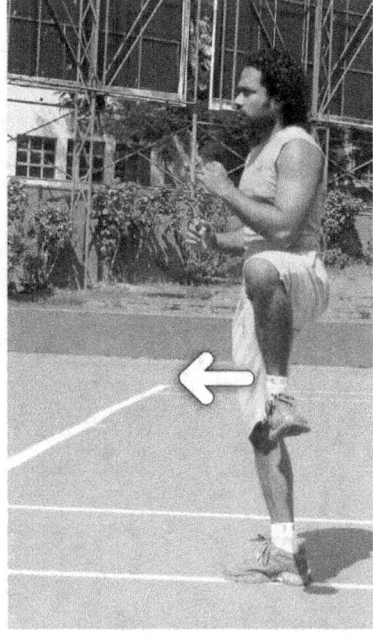

- Start with your feet together and look straight ahead.
- Lift the left leg as seen in the photo and imagine you are moving forward while stepping over hurdles.
- Repeat with right leg.

8) Arm Circles with Forward Steps

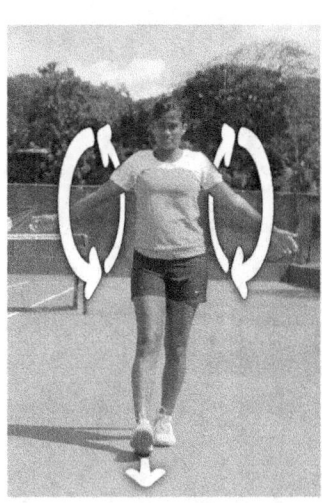 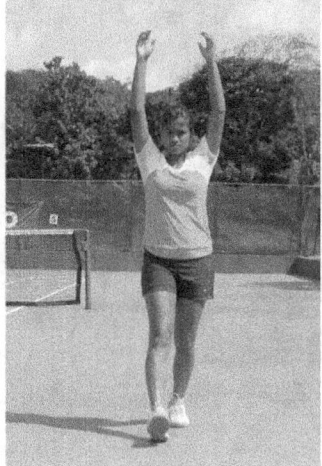

- As you circle your arms backward, point your toes toward the sky.
- As you step with the alternate foot, keep moving your arms and complete a full circle.

9) Arm Circle Forward with Toes Back

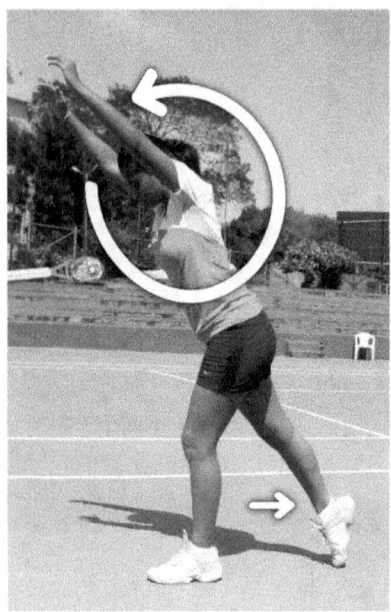

- Step back with the right leg and point toes as shown.
- Angle your body slightly forward, as if you are doing a follow-through after a serve.
- Circle your arms forward while alternating feet.

10) Crossover Lunge

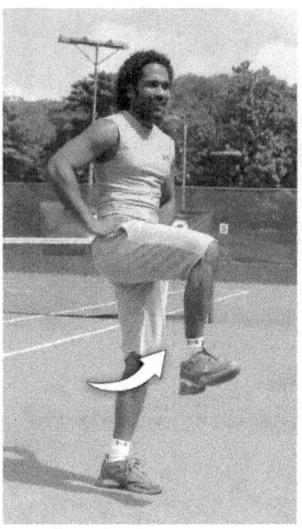 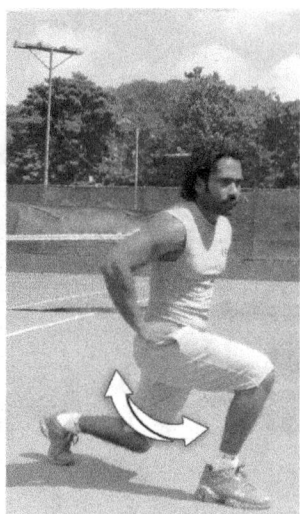

- Start with feet together.
- Raise your right knee to hip level and step across your body to the left as shown.
- Return to the starting position and repeat with your left leg.

SECTION 2—CARDIOVASCULAR FITNESS FOR TENNIS

This is generally referred to as endurance (prolonged activity done at low intensity) or aerobic training using oxygen for the body's energy production).

Benefits of Training with This System
1. Strengthens the muscles involved in respiration (moving oxygen to and from lungs).
2. Enlarges the heart (increases the pumped blood and decreases resting heart rate).
3. Improves circulation and decreases blood pressure.
4. Increases red blood cell count to facilitate transportation of oxygen.
5. High-intensity aerobic training (jogging and running) stimulates bone growth, thereby decreasing the risk of osteoporosis.
6. Increases the blood flow to the muscles.
7. Increases the speed at which aerobic metabolism is activated within muscles. This process allows a greater portion of the energy for intense exercises to be generated aerobically.
8. Improves the ability of muscles to burn fat during exercises, preserving intramuscular glycogen.
9. Enhances the speed at which muscles recover from high-intensity exercise.

Aerobic Capacity (VO2 Max)
If you read fitness articles on the web or in magazines, you may recognize this term. Let's explore it.

VO2 Max refers to the capacity of the cardiorespiratory system (heart, lungs, and blood vessels) and the maximum amount of oxygen the body can use during a specific period of intense exercise. In other words, it has to do with cardiorespiratory performance and the maximum ability to remove and utilize oxygen for circulatory blood.

It's recommend that you maintain around twenty to forty minutes of exercise at an intensity of 60–75 percent of your maximum heart rate at least two to three times per week.

Note that this is a general guideline. Please talk to your fitness professional before deciding the proper zone. It may vary depending on your individual health status, goals, previous exercise habits and other factors.

Cardiovascular Exercises

1. Play basketball on a singles court with a basketball, tennis ball or medicine ball. Use only rotation movements and overhead throws with no breaks.
2. Run around the court while the coach gives different directional cues (forward, side, backward, high knees); do stair runs (up and down).
3. If exercising in a group, call out a name. If alone, call out the names of different objects around the surrounding area.
4. Play soccer over the net on a singles court or basketball court, dribbling the length of half the court.

1) **CV with Basketball, Medicine Ball or Tennis Ball**

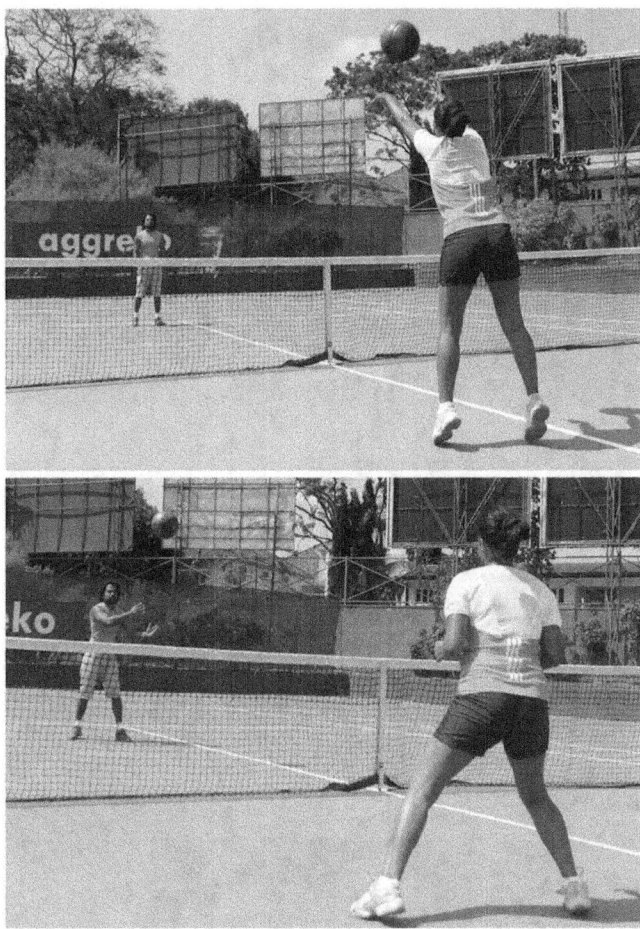

- Face your partner from the opposite side of the court.
- Play on the singles court or the doubles court.
- Throw the ball in a rotational motion from your right side and left side above the net, using both hands. On the opposite side, your partner returns it. Continue to go back and forth.
- Do an overhead throw using both hands.
- The idea is to play nonstop for at least twenty or thirty minutes and try to get points.
- You are only allowed to handle the ball after one bounce or no bounces.

2) CV Stair Runs and Running with Different Cues

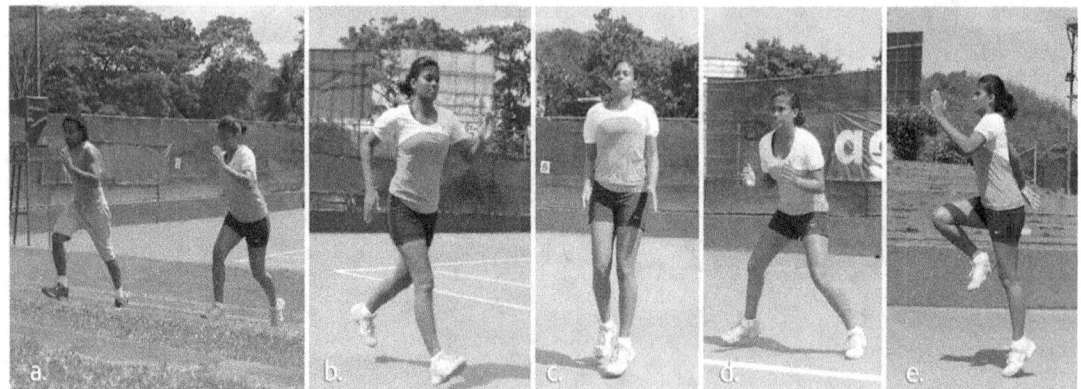

a. Stair runs up and down
b. Running forward
c. Running backward
d. Sidestepping
e. High knees

- For steps *b* through *e*, a coach can command the change of direction or technique.
- Try to maintain a constant phase for thirty to forty-five minutes.

3) Basketball Dribbling and Playing Soccer Over the Net

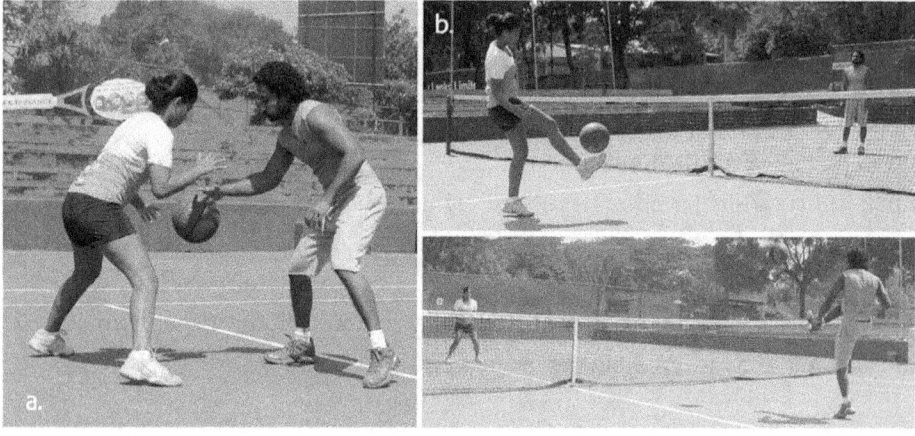

- a) With your partner, use the full court or half court. The idea is to keep moving all the time.
- Try to take the ball from your partner's hand.
- Then dribble the ball, go towards the net, and touch the net with the basketball.
- b) Try to hit and kick a soccer ball over the net.
- Use the singles or doubles court. If you do not get it in one bounce, you will lose the point.

SECTION 3 — STABILITY (BALANCE)

In tennis, stability is required when you set up for a stroke (static stability) or when you move (dynamic stability). Your body must be steady from head to toe and while moving in a linear or angular motion.

Stability is acquired from multiple senses, including hearing, vision, touch, and proprioception (somatosensory).

While the body's motor system controls your muscles, the senses detect changes of body position with respect to the base, regardless of how the body moves or the base moves. In other words, when you lose stability when standing, your body will take corrective action automatically.

Body Weight Stability Training
1) Lower body—both legs, single leg; alternate and add rotation for variety.
2) Upper body—both arms, single arm; alternate and add rotation for variety.

Core Stability Training
Planks, plank single leg, side planks, rotation

Duration: five to ten seconds
Repetitions: Varies upon your requirements
Sets: three to five sets

1) Lower-Body Stability with Both Feet

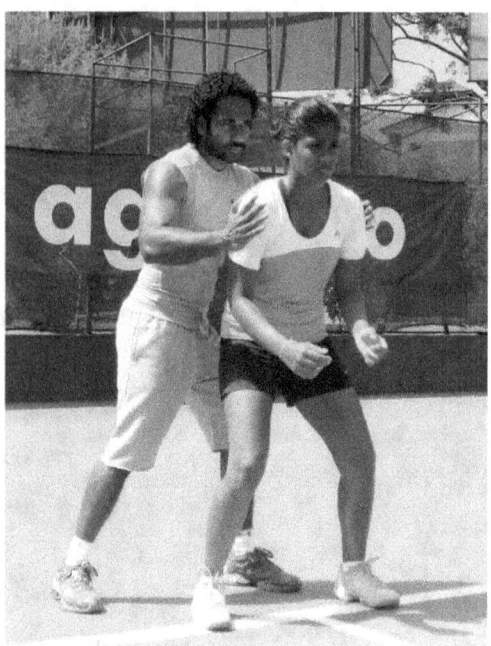

- Ask your student or partner to stand on the baseline with both feet firmly on the court.
- Apply multidirectional forces to make him or her lose balance.

2) Lower-Body Multidirectional Stability

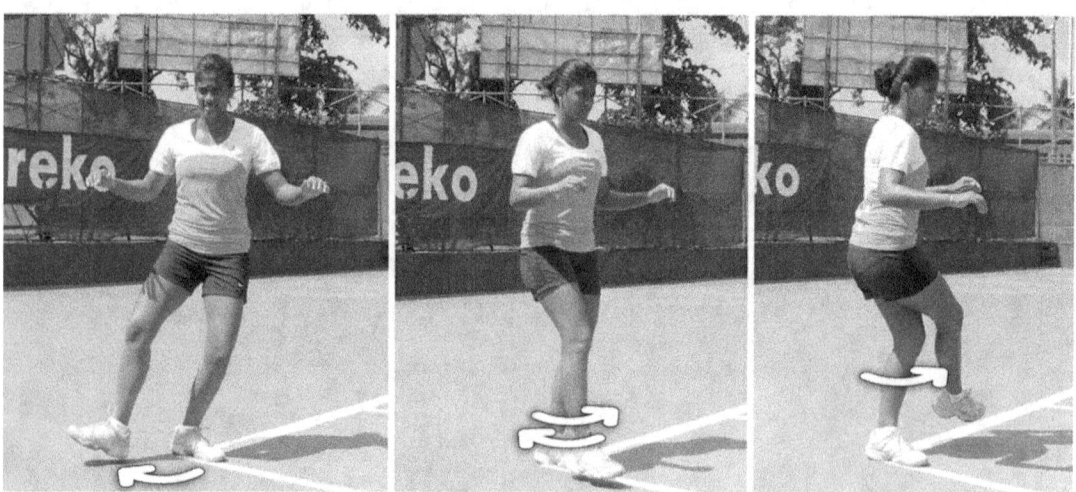

- As shown, first move your left foot to the side, back and forth, and then across.
- This will help you develop good ankle, knee, and hip stability as well as core stability.
- Repeat in all directions several times and then start with the opposite leg.

3) Single-Leg Stability

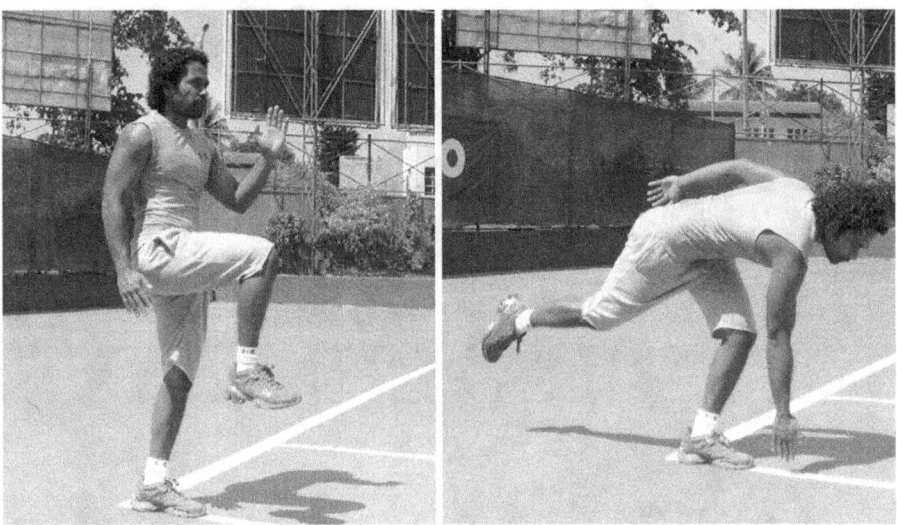

- As shown, start by raising the opposite arm and leg (imagine a runner).
- Reach down, trying to get your right-hand fingers in line with the toes on your left foot.
- Do several repetitions and then repeat on the opposite side.

4) Alternate Dynamic Stability

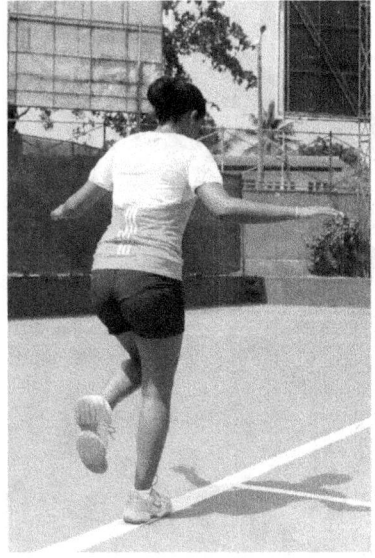

- Stand on the baseline.
- Spread out your arms.
- Take steps with alternating feet.
- Step with right foot, hold for three to five seconds, and then step with the left foot and repeat.

5) Upper-Body Two-Arm Stability

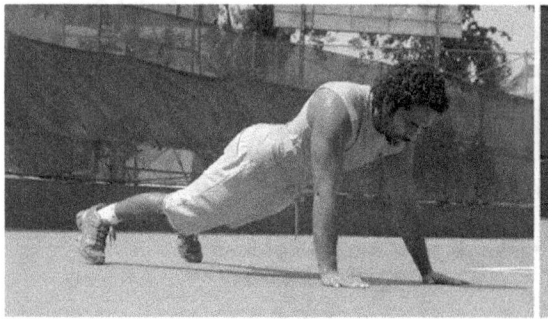 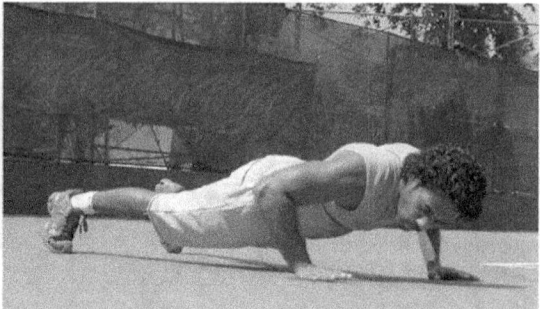

- As shown in the first photo, lock your arms and hold the position.
- For an advanced variation, move down (as in a push-up position) and hold.
- This is a good upper-body stabilization exercise (with emphasis on shoulder stability).

6) Upper-Body Alternate-Arm Stability

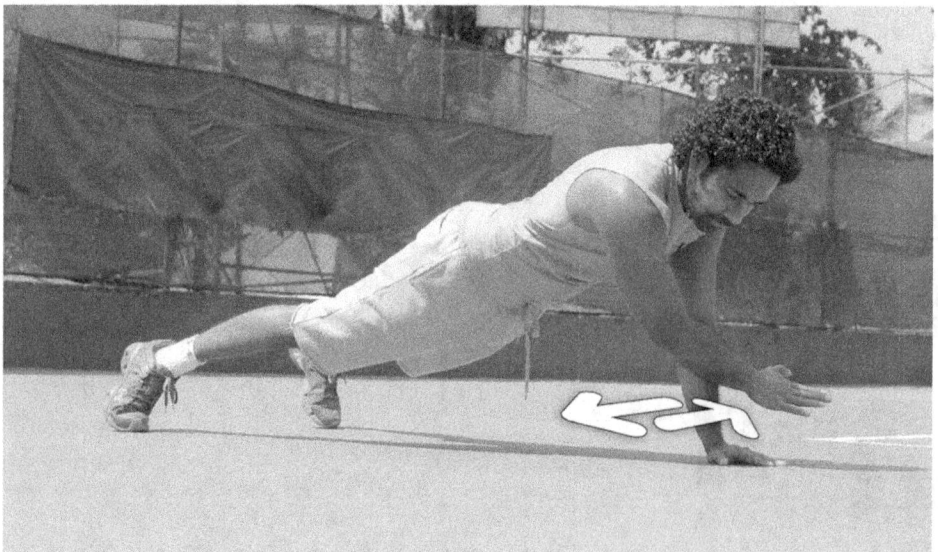

- Keep your arms in the locked position.
- Try to bring your right wrist so that it crosses your left wrist, and then alternate arms.
- This is a good exercise for shoulder and core stability.

7) Single-Arm Stability

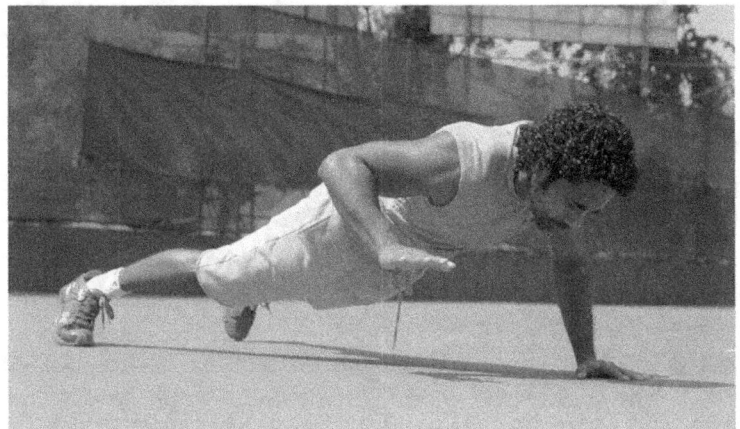

- From a push-up position, lift your right hand (this is an advanced variation).
- This will give you greater challenge for increasing wrist, elbow, and shoulder stability.
- This focuses on your core stability as well.

8) Core Stability

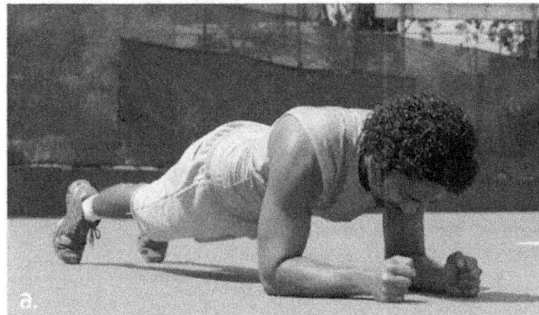 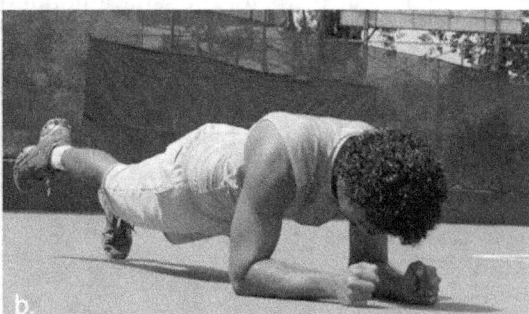

- Keep your forearm rested on the floor with the elbow in line with shoulders and keep your abdominals tight and in a straight line.
- The stance shown in image *a* is one of the best abdominal stability exercises.
- Image *b* shows an advanced progression that gives a greater challenge to your core. This can be achieved by lifting one foot off the ground and then changing feet after the intended time.
- Make sure you do not arch your back when performing this exercise.
- You can also do a beginner version by placing your knees on the ground.

9) Core Side Plank

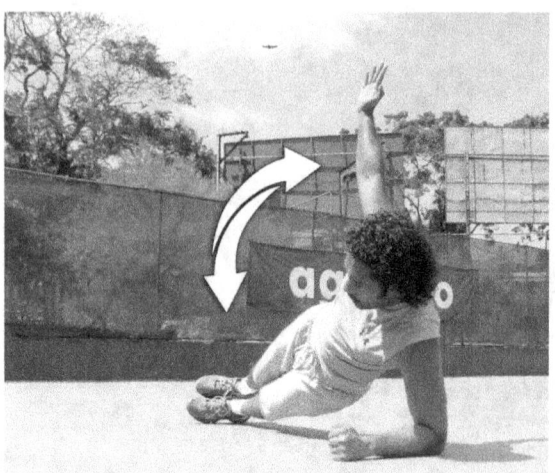

- Start by lying on either your left side or right side.
- Slightly lift your body as shown above and hold the position.
- Beginners may rest their right hand on their right thigh.
- As you progress, you can lift your hand as shown in the photo.
- Hold the side plank for the same amount of time on the other side of your body as well.

10) Upper-Body Rotational

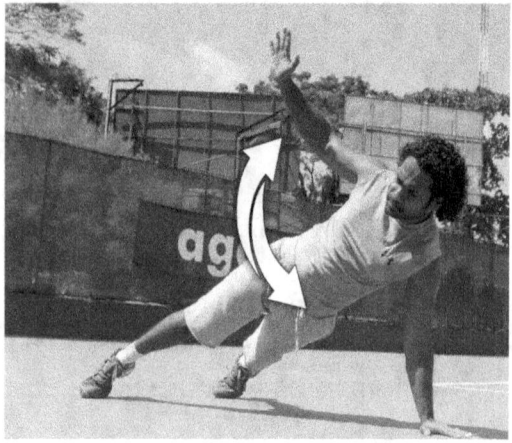

- Depending on your fitness level, you can start in a push-up position or a lockout position refer 5) on Upper body two arm stability position.
- You can then rotate your entire body to the right side or the left side for several repetitions.
- As you progress, you can do alternate sides. This will enhance your rotational acceleration, deceleration with stabilization and transferring of weight bearing from your left arm to right arm.
- This is an exercise for total-body coordinated movement with stability.

SECTION 4—COORDINATION

In your daily activity, your body needs to contract and move in a synchronized manner. Hence proper movement is made up of proper timing, speed, and intensity.

This combination runs from head to toe and is widely known in the strength and conditioning field and sports communities as a "coordination chain" or "kinetic chain."

This concept means that the force from one link transfers to the next link (e.g., lower leg, upper leg, torso, upper body, arms) from the ground upward, as in a tennis serve.

Any activity which requires technique and skill can improve in the five areas below, which are the key components of coordination.

a) **Orientation**: To gauge and modify movement in space, allowing time for action (e.g., a lob in tennis).

b) **Differentiation**: The ability to control internal and external information and use it in your daily life or the sport you play (e.g., return of serve).

c) **Stability**: Having total awareness of your body and surroundings will give you good balance, increasing your court movement in multidirectional running and helping you set up and produce a powerful stroke.

d) **Reaction**: Reacting to simple or complex actions by opponents (e.g., high- or low-speed rallies or countering a high-speed serve). For example, when you are relaxing on the beach and you see a huge wave is in your path, many would try to move away as soon as possible.

e) **Rhythm**: Maintaining proper timing will give you fluidity in motion.

If you consider the top ten male and female tennis players in the world, you will notice their rhythm when they step on to the court. Figure skaters, dancers, and soccer players also demonstrate this ability. If you lose your rhythm, the opponent will take advantage of it. Note that it varies from sport to sport.

Hand-eye, foot-eye, and total body coordination are the categories discussed most often.

1) Foot-Eye Coordination

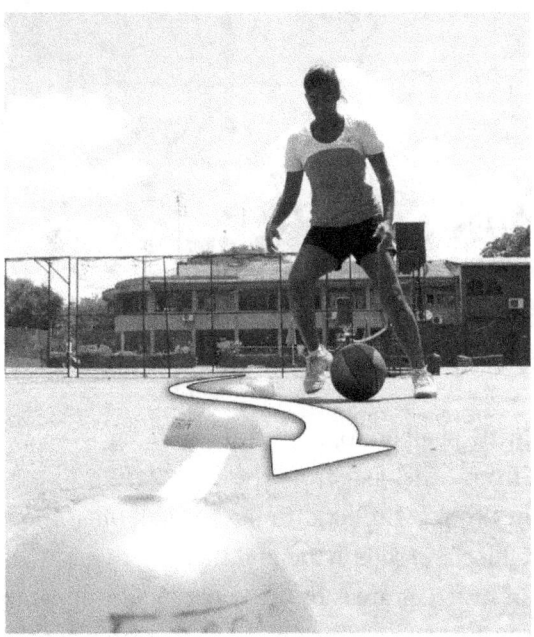

- Use a soccer ball or tennis ball.
- Set up cones in a straight line or in various directions. Using only your feet, try to maneuver the ball without hitting the cones/targets.

2) Hand-Eye Coordination

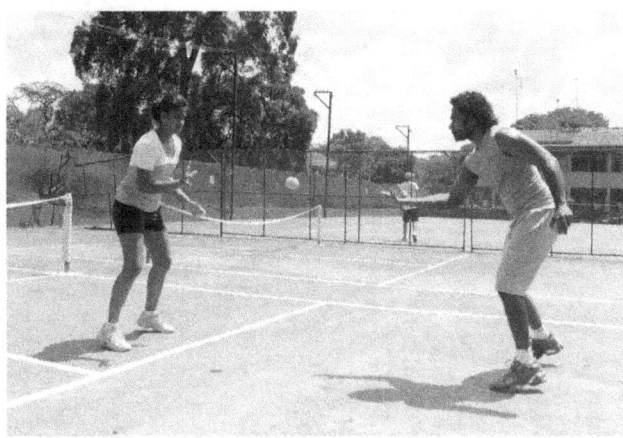

- Stand facing your partner.
- Throw the tennis ball back and forth to each other. You can catch with either hand.
- The catcher must respond to the verbal and visual cues from the thrower (e.g., right to right or left to right).

3) Total Body Coordination

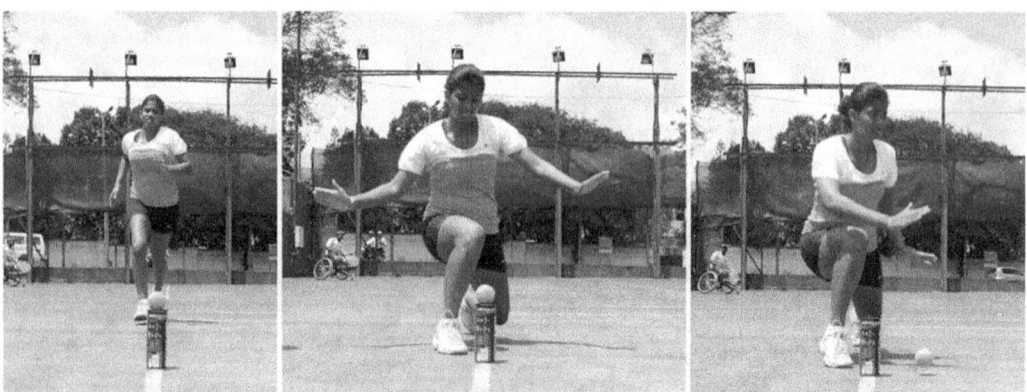

- Place a ball can in the center of the baseline with a ball on top.
- On your partner's command, run to the can from either side from the doubles line.
- As shown, bend using the right leg and swing your right hand to tap the ball off without moving the can itself. For variety, use your left leg and right hand and then alternate.
- For an advanced version, place many cans in different areas of the court. Following your partner's cues, run toward a particular can and hit the ball, pick up the ball, or replace the ball without moving the can.

4) Dribbling a Basketball or Tennis Ball

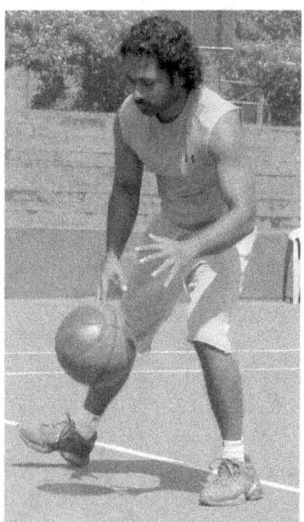

- Following instructions from your partner or coach dribble the ball using only your right hand, only your left hand or alternate hands.
- Use forward movement, backward movement, and side movements to create your own combination (e.g., three steps forward, five steps backward, two steps right, and one step left).

SECTION 5—MUSCLE SIZE, STRENGTH, ENDURANCE, AND POWER

Muscles are an integral part of movement. To develop your muscles, you can do strength training. Specifically, resistance training builds the endurance, size, strength, and power of your muscles; your nervous system and bones also adapt. Gravity, body weights, elastic or rubber bands, dumbbells, barbells, water, and many more are common tools for strength training. In this book, we will cover dumbbells, elastic and rubber tubing, and medicine balls to contract muscles for different goals.

Benefits of Strength and Resistance Training
   a) Increases strength in bones, muscles, tendons (connecting muscle to bone), and ligaments (connecting bone to bone).
   b) Increases joint function, decreases potential injury, and increases bone density and metabolism.
   c) Increases heart function and good cholesterol (HDL).
   d) Strength training is anaerobic in nature; however, if you incorporate circuit training, it will give you some aerobic benefits as well.

Strength training may vary depending on your individual goals or the sport you are playing. It must be organized by a trained fitness professional. However, everyone could benefit from endurance training and hypertrophy training.

My athletes and clients often ask about the difference between elastic or rubber tubing and free weights.
   A) Using free weights, such as dumbbells and barbells provides the majority of resistance to the joint when the movement begins and when the muscle overcomes inertia.
   B) Elastic tubing gives the greatest contraction at the end of the movement. To enhance your progress, it is best to utilize both these methods with other methods so that your body will

adapt to various types of equipment, tension, and speed. Therefore, you shouldn't stick to a single training program.

Remember that the angle of a joint can alter the force you produce, as force depends on leverage.

There are some commonly used terminologies in resistance training. These can also be used in the areas of speed, agility, cardiovascular training etc.

a) Concentric contraction: muscle shortens against resistance.
b) Eccentric contraction: muscle lengthens against resistance.
c) Isometric contraction: muscle length stays static at a particular angle against resistance.
d) Reps (repetitions): lifting and lowering multiple times.
e) Sets: the number of reps (depends on your goals).
f) Rest: a rest between sets or exercises to gain the maximum results.
g) Speed (tempo): depends on the goal you're trying to reach.

The focus of this book is to provide an affordable workout that requires less equipment but provides a good fitness base, whether for health and fitness purposes or as a foundation for more competitive tennis.

If you plan to play in tournaments, it's highly advisable that you find a certified strength coach, performance coach or a trainer. The difference between winning and losing comes from selecting proper exercises, planning your tournament calendar, incorporating progress and the appropriate fitness components as well as strength, power endurance (power in a fatigue stage), rest, nutrition etc.

Professional players have a medical team that includes a nutritionist, a physical therapist, a tennis coach, and a performance coach. The Internet and books will not help you get the same results as pro players. Professional results will only be in your grasp if you team up with the good team of professionals.

However, the following guidelines will help you train efficiently.

1) **Basic Conditioning**
   This provides the ability to perform with a high level of force for a prolonged period of time.
   a) Muscle endurance—a low intensity activity with a high number of reps and decreased resting time (12–20 reps)
   b) Strength endurance—a higher level of force with fewer reps (8–12)

Reps: 8–12 or 12–20 (depending on your goals and training level)
Sets: 2–4
Rest: 1 minute
Tempo: moderately fast
Frequency: 2–4 times per week

2) Hypertrophy

Increases the size (volume) of a single muscle or multiple muscles.
Reps: 8–12
Sets: 3–5
Rest: 1–2 minutes
Tempo: moderate to slow
Frequency: 3–6 times per week

3) Strength Training

Training to increase the maximum force a muscle can produce in a single voluntary effort.

Reps: 1–5
Sets: 4–6
Rest: 3–5 minutes
Tempo: fast
Frequency: 2–4 times per week

4) Power

The ability of the nerves and muscles to produce the greatest possible force in the shortest time period. Strength combined with speed creates power.

Power training can set the platform for advanced training methods such as power endurance and producing high power in a fatigue stage. As a tennis player, it is ideal to use multi-joint exercises.

Reps: 1–5
Sets: 3–5
Rest: 2–6 minutes
Tempo: fast as possible (with good form)
Frequency: 2–4 times per week

5) Power Endurance

This type of training produces high-power, activity-specific movement in a fatigue stage. For example, in tennis, it simulates a rally with the proper rest time between making a point and continuing.

This should be administered by your strength and conditioning or performance coach and only for competitive players with a good fitness base.

Note: All exercises are grouped in muscles and can be manipulated using the above suggestions, according to your training goals.

Legs

1) Band Squat

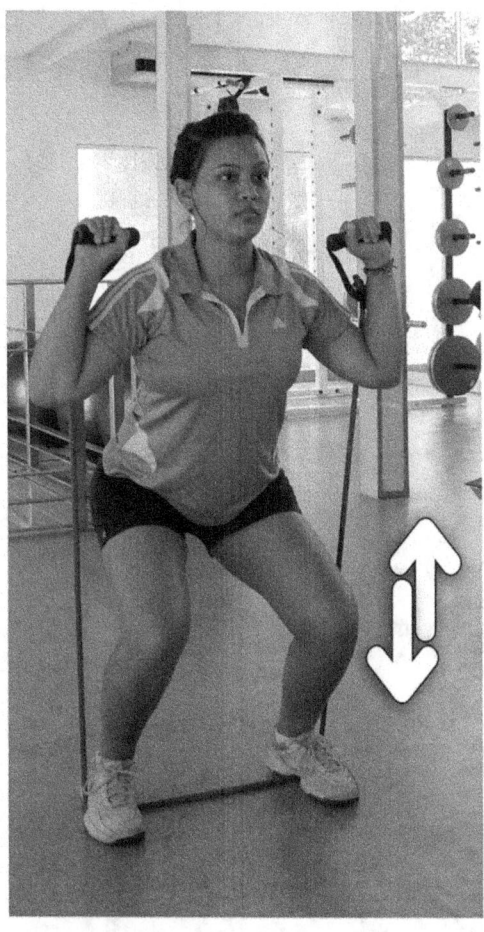

- Start with the ends of the band at your sides and behind your back, with your palms at shoulder level.
- Squat down so that your thighs are almost parallel to the floor.
- Contract your leg muscles and come up so that your knees are in a lockout position.

2) Band Lunge

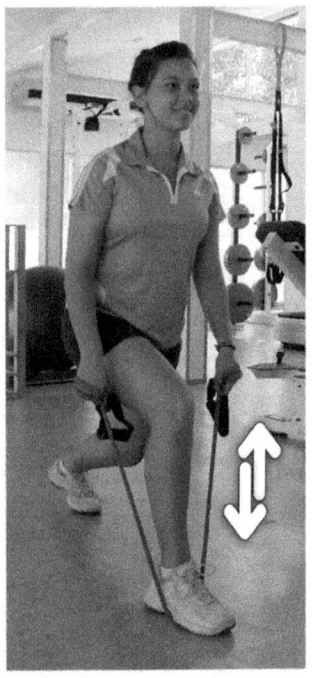

- Hold the ends of the band on either side of your body and keep your right foot in front.
- Maintain an upright position as shown.
- Lower yourself so that your knee is bent at a 90-degree angle.
- Come up as you contract your leg muscle. Change legs and repeat.

3) Ball Hamstring Curl

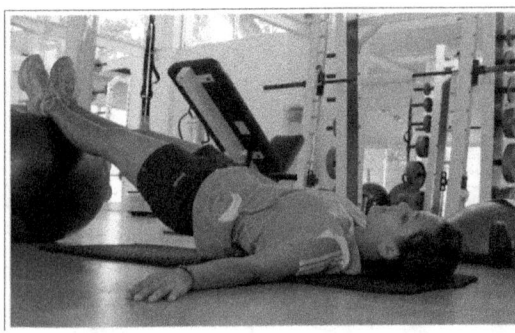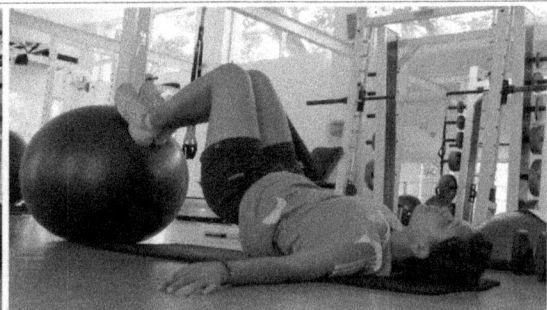

- Rest your heels on the stability ball.
- Lift your buttocks while keeping your palms facedown, pressing against the floor.
- By maintaining this position, you can curl the ball back and forth.
- This is a great exercise for the back of your thighs to strengthen the hamstrings.

4) Dumbbell Squat

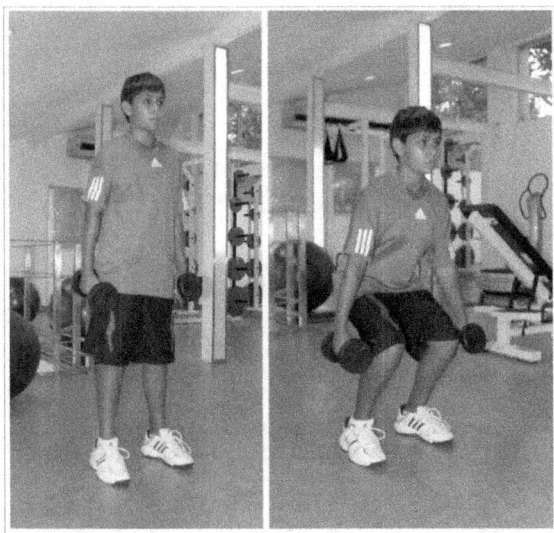

- Hold the dumbbells by your sides.
- Visualize that you are sitting on a chair and try to move your buttocks toward that imaginary chair.
- Contract the muscle as you come back to the starting position.

5) Dumbbell Lunge

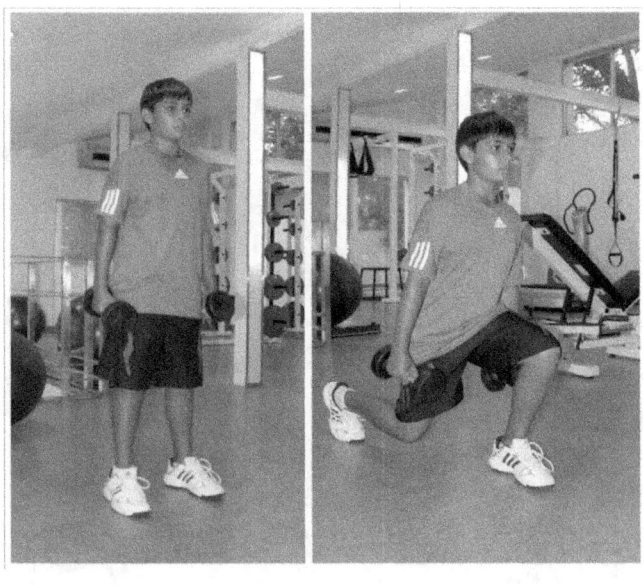

- From a standing position, take a step forward and lunge either from your right or left foot and come back to the starting position.
- Repeat from the same leg or the other leg by alternating, keeping your hands by your sides. The idea is to reach forward.
- Beginners may start from a standing position and try to step backward instead of forward.

6) Dumbbell Side Lunge

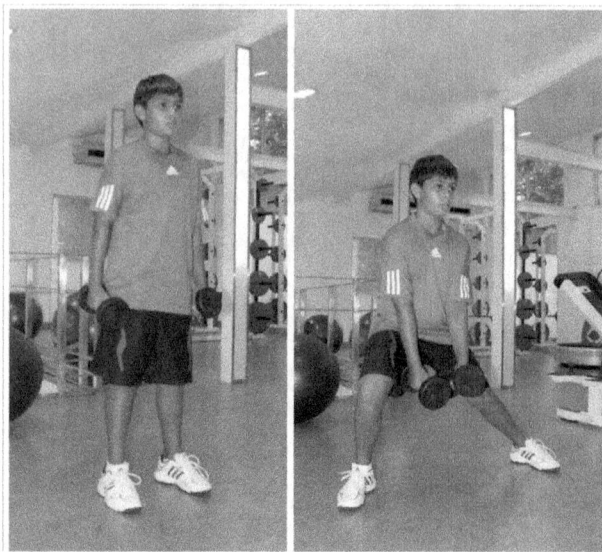

- From a standing position, hold the dumbbells by your sides or in front of your body.
- Take a side step to the right, as shown.
- Come back to the starting position and repeat on the left side.
- You can complete all your reps on one side first or do it on alternate sides.

7) Dumbbell Rotation Lunge

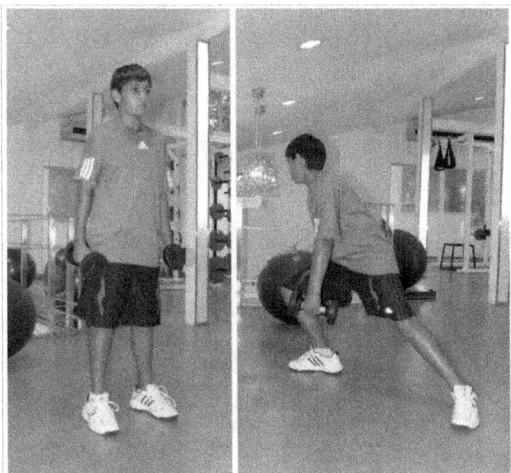

- From a standing position (visualize standing facing 12 o'clock and you rotate back to a 5 o'clock if using the right leg or 7 o'clock if using the left leg. Take your right leg and rotate backward as you complete the lunge.
- Return to the starting position and repeat on the opposite side.
- Reps can be performed one leg at a time or on alternate legs.

8) Dumbbell Dead Lift (Straight Leg)

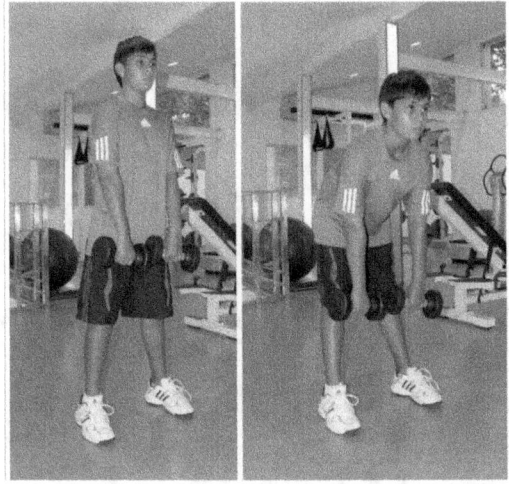

- Hold the weights in front of your body.
- Try to lower the dumbbells until they reach slightly below your knees.
- When performing this exercise, keep your knees slightly bent, your stomach pulled in, and your back as straight as possible without arching it.
- Return to the starting position and repeat.

9) Dumbbell Calves

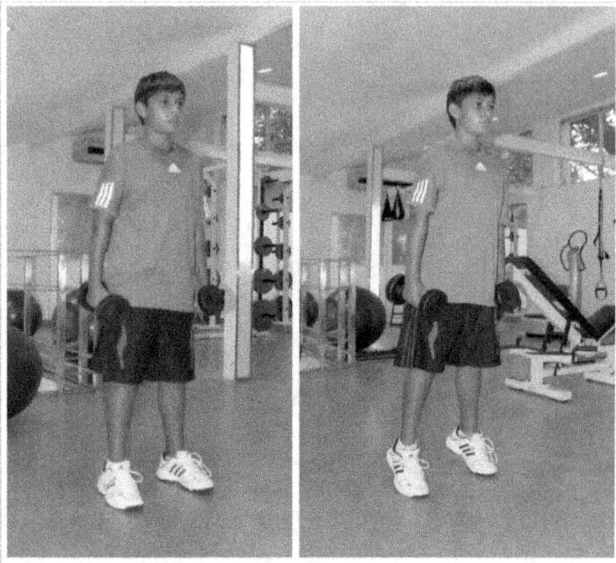

- From a standing position, transfer the weight to the balls of your feet and raise your heels.
- Return to the starting position, placing your heels back down on the floor.
- You can repeat this exercise with variations, such as using a single leg or alternating legs.

10) Squat Jump (Power)

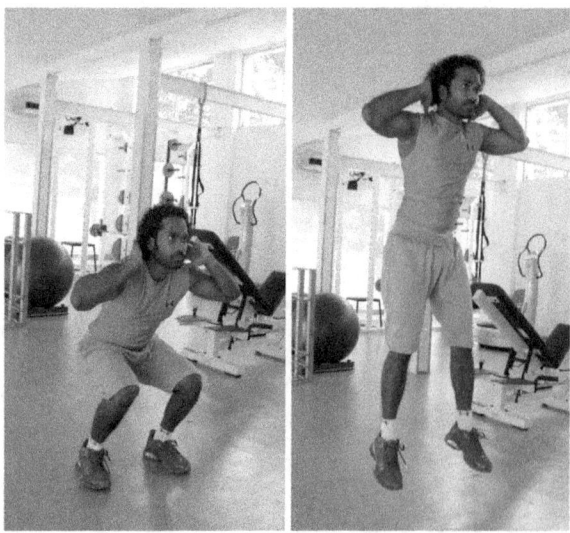

- Start with feet shoulder-width apart and arms behind your head.
- Squat to a 90 degree angle so that your thighs are parallel to the floor.
- Put your weight on your legs and jump up on a vertical line.

11) Lunge Jumps (Power)

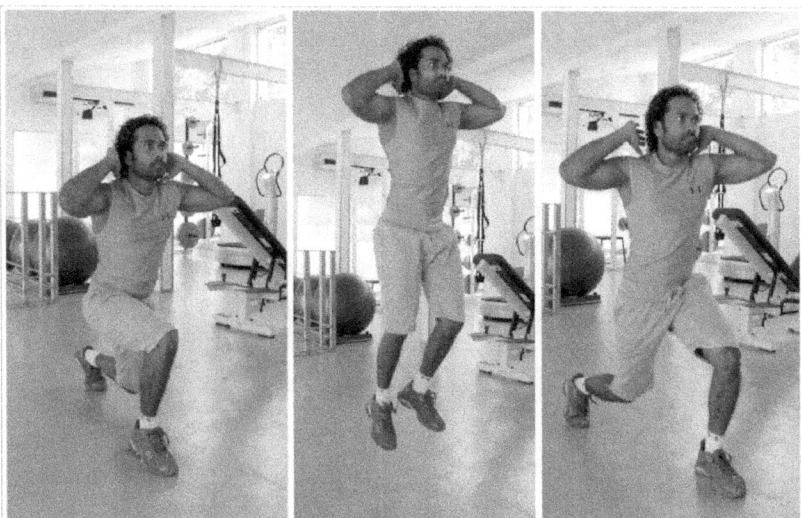

- Start by placing your hands behind your head while in a lunge position.
- As you propel yourself upward, switch feet in the air (as shown in the middle photo) and land on the opposite foot from the one you started with.
- Lower yourself into the lunge position and repeat.

12) Calf Jumps (Power)

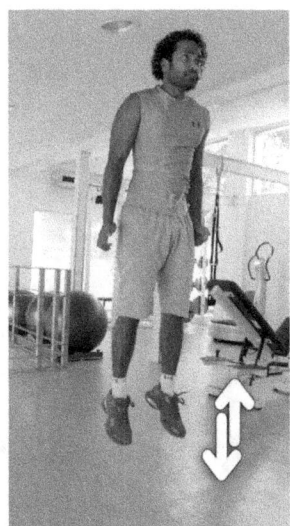

- From a standing position, maintain slightly locked knees.
- Use the balls of your feet to project yourself upward.
- Repeat.

13) Box Jump (Power)

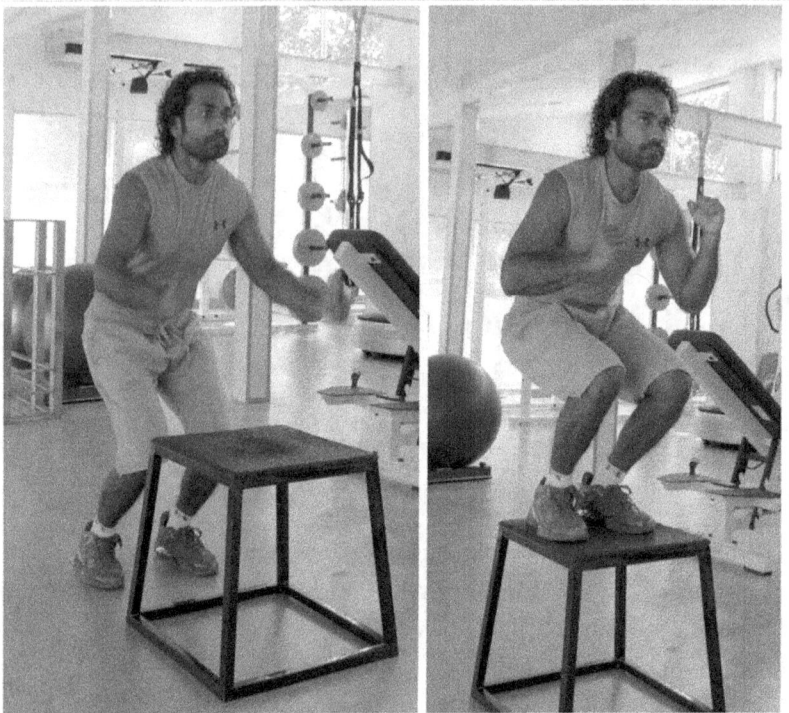

- From a slight squatting position, preload your muscles and jump onto the box with both feet.
- Return to the starting position by stepping down or jumping down, depending on your level of fitness and performance.

Chest

1) Band Chest Fly

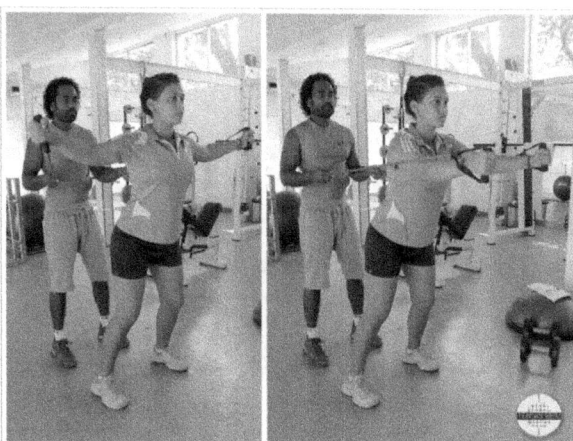

- Start with your arms apart and knees slightly bent. Hold your body upright as shown.
- Contracting the chest muscles, bring your palms together in front of your body.
- Return to the starting position slowly.

2) Band Chest Press

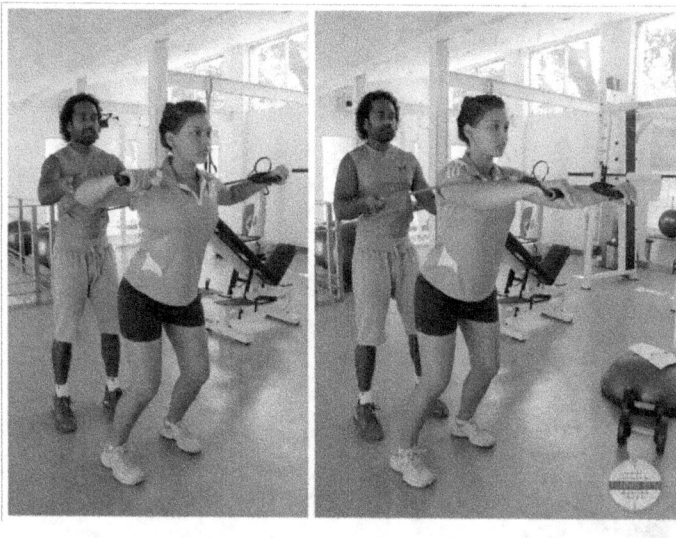

- Start in an upright position with knees slightly bent.
- Hold elbows at a 90-degree angle, with your palms facing down, in line with your chest.
- Contracting the chest muscles, press your arms forward so that the bands and arms come to the center of your chest. (visualize pushing a cabinet)
- Slowly return your hands to the starting position and repeat.

3) Band Chest Rotation

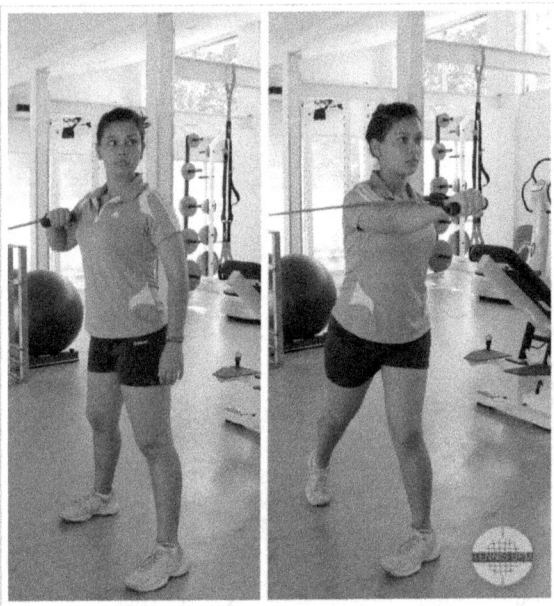

- As shown in the first photo, keep your right hand in line with the right side of your chest.
- Pivot your right foot as you press your right hand across your chest.
- Make sure your left foot remains still.
- Return to the starting position slowly and repeat.
- Change sides after you complete the recommended number of sets and reps.

4) Ball Push-Up

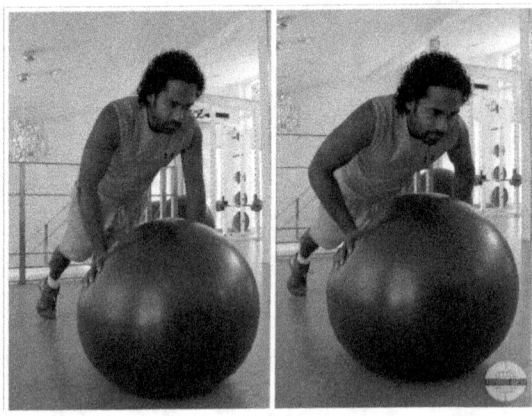

- Place your hands on the stability ball and maintain a straight body position.
- Drop your body forward in a controlled movement and come back to the starting position.
- As an advanced variation, you can progress to this exercise by starting in a bent-knee position on the floor with your hands on the ball.

5) Floor Push-Up

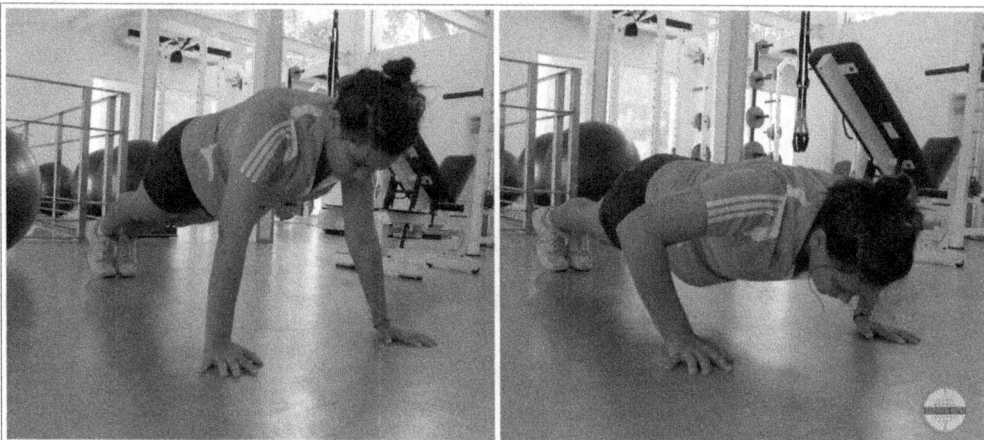

- Start with your palms on the floor at shoulder width, your body straight, and your feet together (keep your feet apart to do a less advanced variation on the exercise).
- Maintaining the position, lower your body so that you come to a position with your elbows bent at a 90-degree angle.
- Return to the starting position, by contracting the chest muscles, and repeat.

6) Dumbbell Hugs

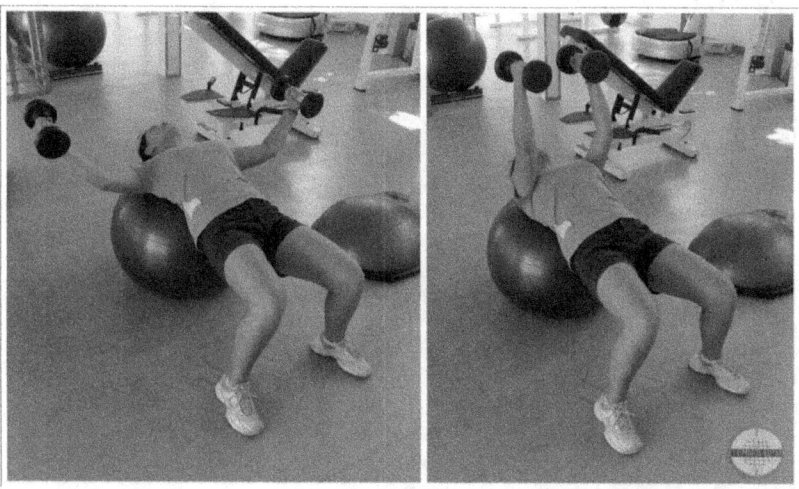

- Start with your upper back resting on the stability ball and your hips raised and parallel to the floor.
- From an open-arm position with elbows slightly bent and palms facing toward each other, bring your arms together in front of your body as you contract the chest muscles, as shown in the photograph.
- Return to the starting position slowly and repeat.

7) Dumbbell Chest Press

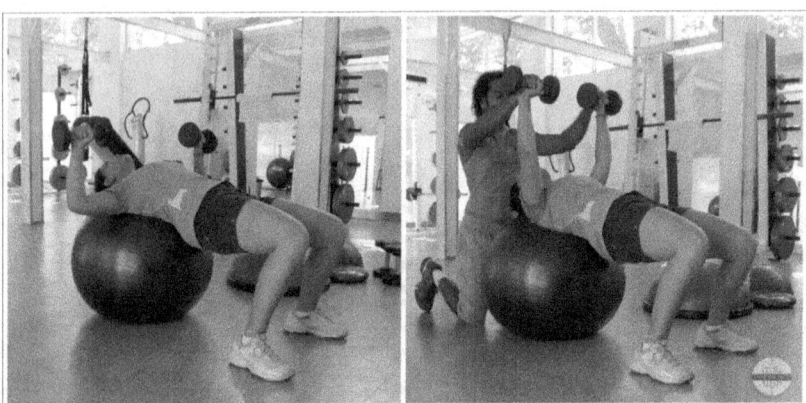

- Start with your upper back resting on the stability ball and your hips raised and parallel to the floor.
- From an open-arm position with elbows bent at 90 degrees and palms facing outward (pic.1), bring your arms together in front of your body as you contract the chest muscles (pic. 2).
- Return to the starting position slowly and repeat. You can ask your partner or coach to spot your movement as shown in photo 2.

8) Medicine Ball Chest Pass (Power)

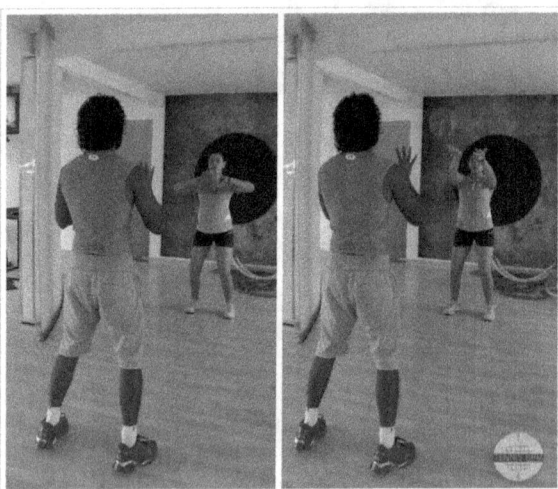

- Stand in an athletic position with bent knees, holding a medicine ball close to your chest.
- Throw the medicine ball at your partner or coach explosively and repeat.
- A modern rubberized medicine ball can be thrown against the type of wall shown in the background of the photo. The black circle is called a wall strike zone.

9) **Medicine Ball Rotational Pass (Power)**

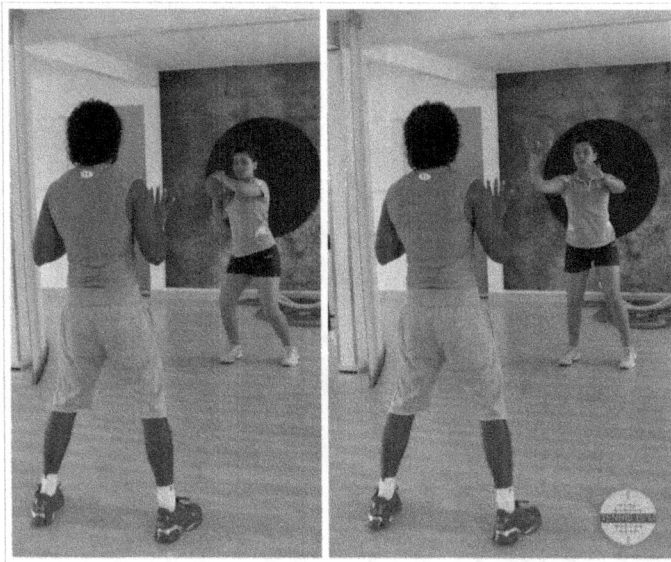

- Start with bent knees and preload the right side of the body, keeping the ball in line with your right chest.
- Explosively release the ball as you rotate. You can increase the angle of rotation as you progress to a total body rotation. A basic level of rotation is shown in the photo.

Back

1) Band High Pull

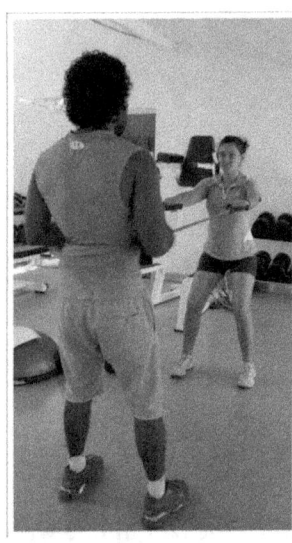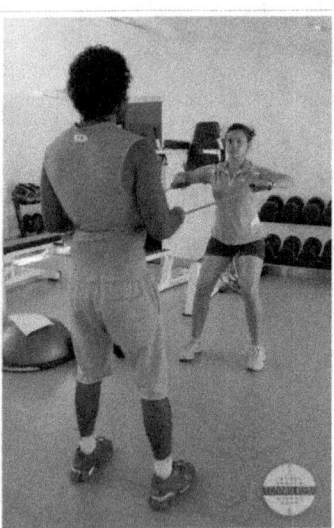

- Start with knees slightly bent and palms gripping the handles at shoulder height.
- Pull your elbows back as you contract the upper back muscles as shown in photo 2.
- Return to the starting position and repeat.

2) Band Low Pull

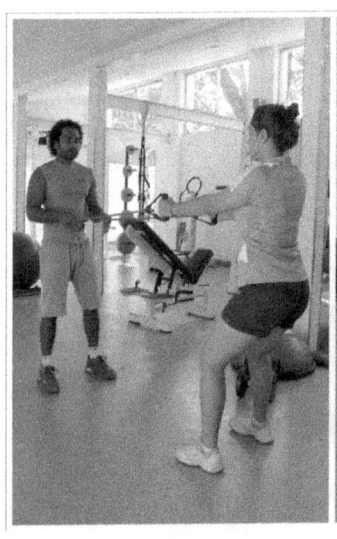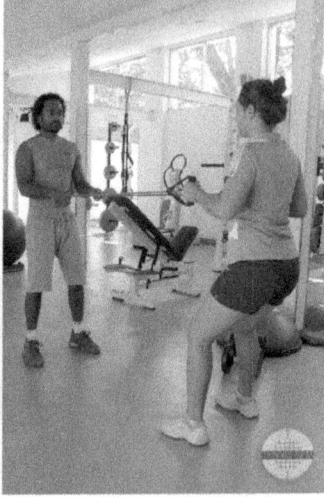

- Start with a bent-knee position with palms slightly lower than shoulder level as shown in photo 1.
- Pull your elbows back by contracting the mid-back muscles as shown in photo 2.
- Return to the starting position and repeat.

3) Band Rotation Backward

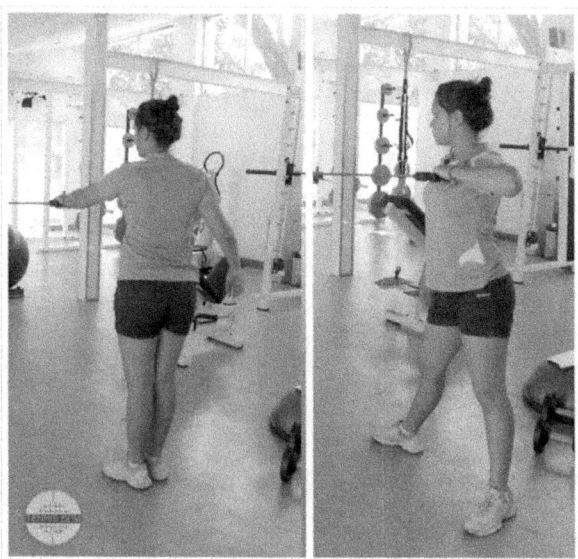

- Stand with your feet together and hold the band with your left hand.
- Keep your right leg stable and pivot your left leg back while you pull the band as shown in photo 2.
- Return to the starting position and repeat on both sides.

4) Body Weight Back Exercise (Pull Ups)

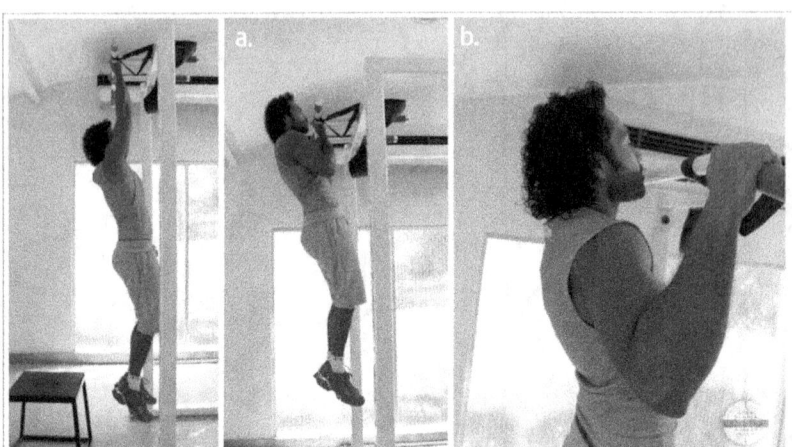

- This is an advanced exercise. It should only be performed under the supervision of a qualified professional.
- Start in a position hanging from the bar and use an underhanded grip as shown in photo *a* or an overhanded grip as shown in photo *b*.
- Your goal is to pull yourself up, contracting the upper, middle, and lower back muscles. Aim to get your chin in line with the bar and eventually passing the bar.
- Gradually lower yourself back to the starting position.
- Once you master this exercise, it is excellent for your back, wrists, forearms, and shoulder strength and stability. Remember that it should only be attempted after proper progression from basic exercises.

5) **Dumbbell Reverse Fly**

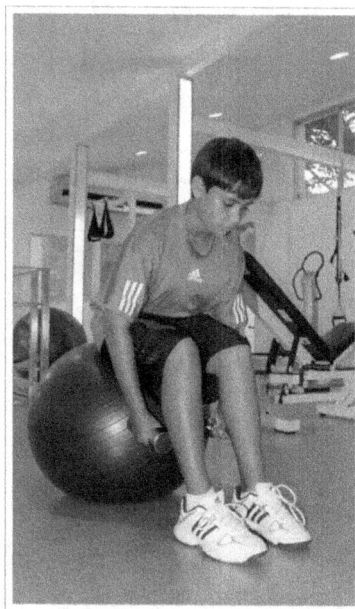 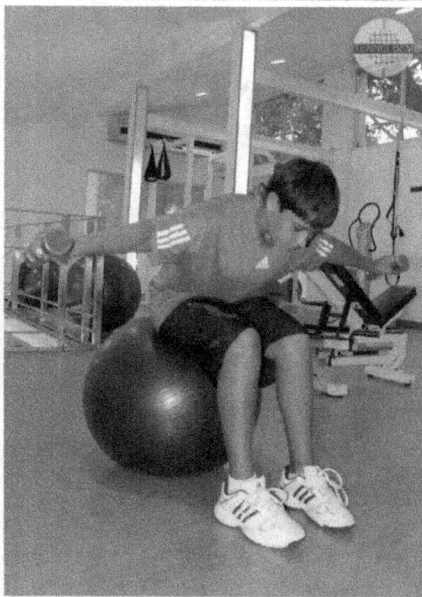

- Sit on a bench or stability ball with your upper body leaning forward as shown in the photo 1.
- Keeping your elbows slightly bent, raise your arms to shoulder level.
- Slowly return to the starting position and repeat.

6) Dumbbell Close Pull

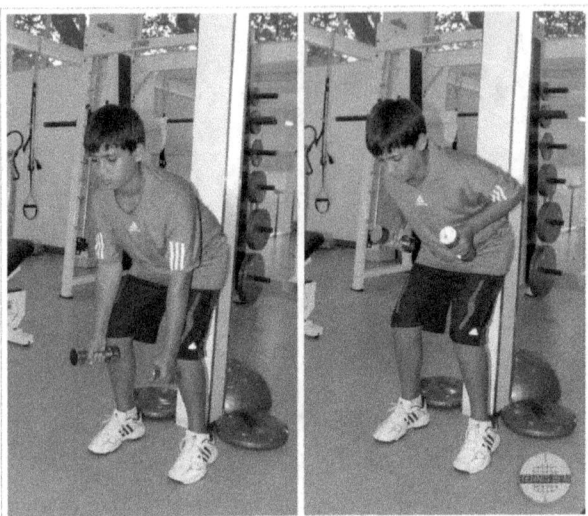

- Start by resting your buttocks on a wall or pillar, keeping your knees slightly bent as you lean forward from your hips. Maintain a straight back and lower your arms as shown in photo 1.
- Pull your elbow up as you contract the back muscles as shown photo 2.
- Return to the starting position and repeat.

7) Dumbbell Upright Row

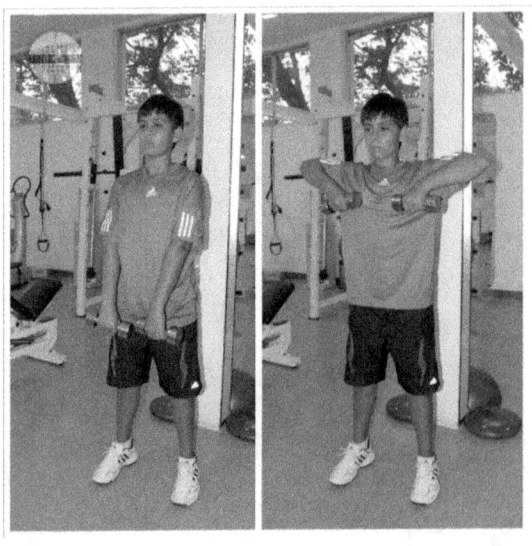

- Stand straight, with your arms in front of your body and your knuckles facing the floor.
- Slowly pull the weight upward, in line with the front of your body as you maintain a downward knuckle position.
- At the end of the motion, elbows will be pointing outward as shown in photo 2.
- Make sure to contract your upper back muscles.
- Return to the starting position and repeat.

8) Medicine Ball Floor Slam (Power)

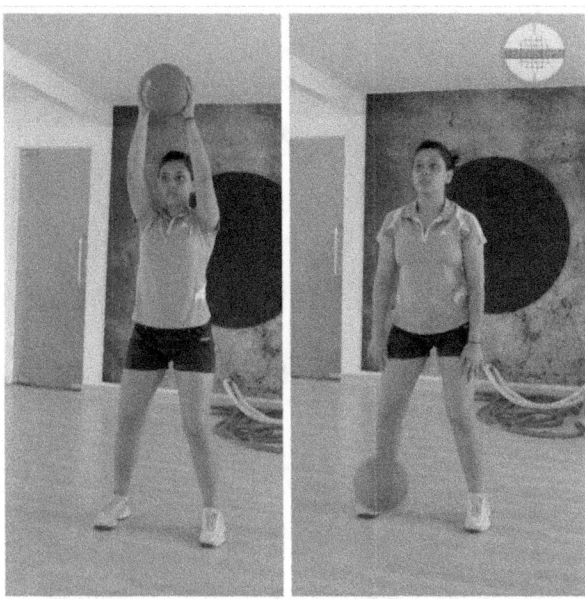

- Stand with bent knees and hold the medicine ball over your head.
- Slam the ball on the floor explosively, as hard and fast as you can, by keeping your arms straight and contracting your back muscles and upper-body side muscles (lats).
- Repeat the exercise.

Arms

1) Arms Band (Bicep)

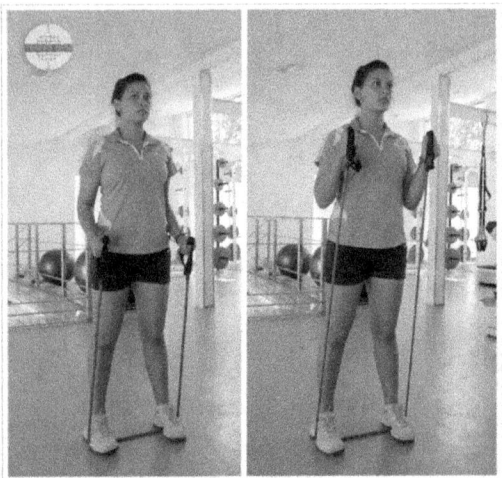

- Start with a slightly flexed elbow so that you can feel the tension of the band (photo 1).
- Contract your arm muscles as you bring them up to shoulder level.
- Make sure your thumb is pointing toward the ceiling (photo 2)
- Return to the starting position and repeat.

2) Band Triceps

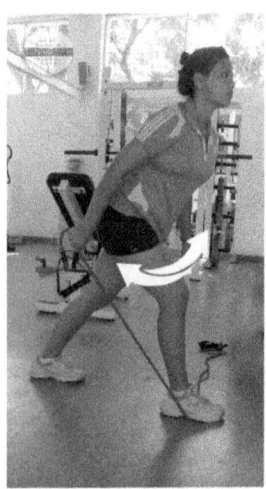

- Start with your elbows bent at hip level.
- As shown in the photo, extend one arm to the end of its range of motion.
- Follow the arrows and repeat the motion.
- At the end of the motion, contract the back arm muscle (triceps) and repeat the exercise.

3) Box Dips

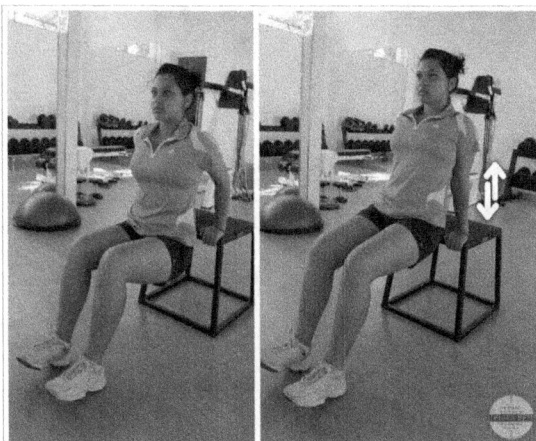

- Start by keeping your knees and elbows at a 90-degree angle with your back straight.
- As you press your palms against the box, extend your elbows by contracting your muscles on the back of your upper arm (triceps).
- Follow the arrows in the photos and repeat.

4) Dumbbell Hammer Curls

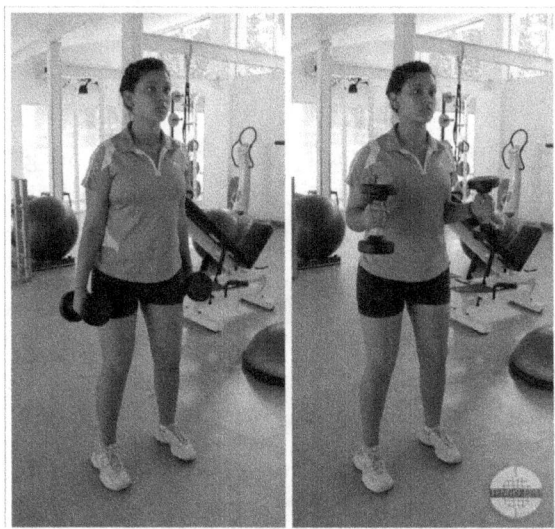

- Start with arms by your sides.
- As you contract the muscles, bring your arms up as shown in photo 2.
- Lower the weight and repeat the motion.

5) Dumbbell Triceps Extension

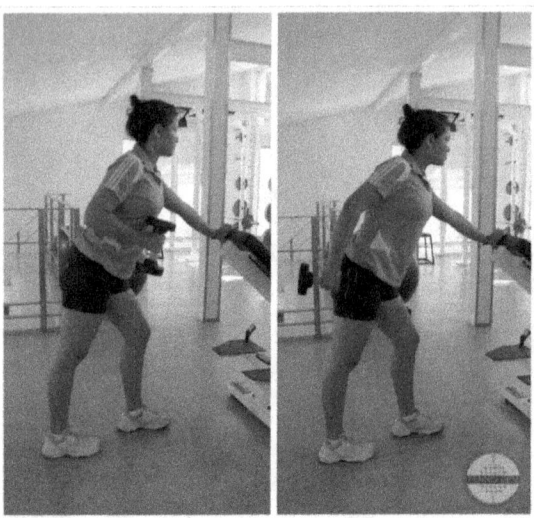

- Start with your arms at 90 degrees and a slightly angled body. Use your non-weight-bearing hand to hold a bench for support.
- As you contract the muscle, extend your arms so that the weight passes to the right thigh as shown in photo 2.
- Complete the exercise on both sides.

6) Forearm Flexion

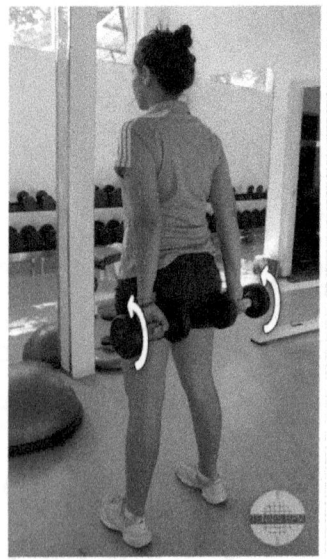

- Start with your knuckles facing the floor and the weight held behind your back as shown in the photo.
- Maintaining your grip on the bars, lift your knuckles up as shown with arrows.
- Return to the starting position and repeat.

7) Forearm Extension

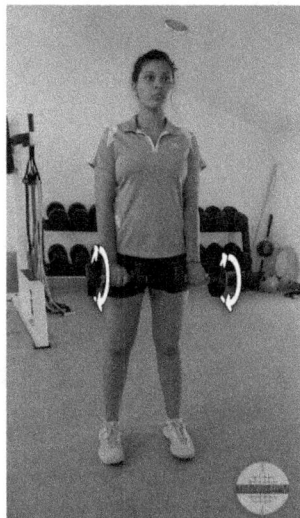

- Start by holding the dumbbells in front of your body with your knuckles facing down.
- As you contract the upper-arm muscles, bring your knuckles upward as shown in photo.
- Return to the starting position and repeat. Follow the arrows in the photo.

8) Medicine Ball Triceps Throw (Power)

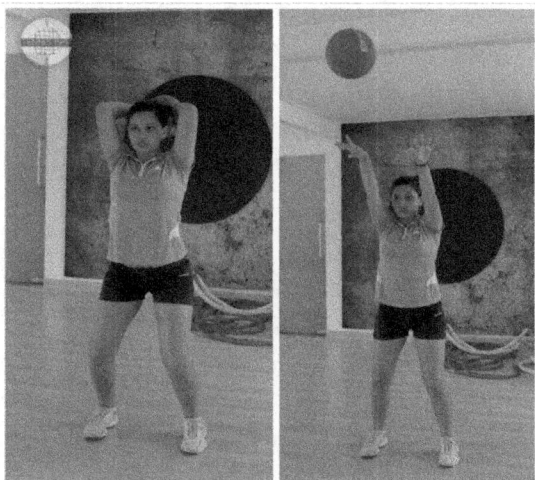

- Start with bent knees, holding the ball behind your head and pointing your elbows forward.
- Explosively throw the ball hard and as fast as you can by contracting your arm muscles.
- Repeat the movements.

Shoulders

1) Band Shoulder Press

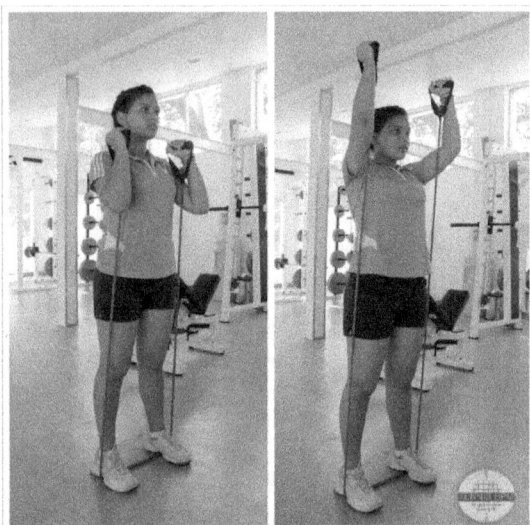

- Start with your arms at shoulder level and your elbows pointing forward.
- Gradually press the arms upward as shown in photo 2.
- Return to the starting position and repeat.

2) Band Wide Press

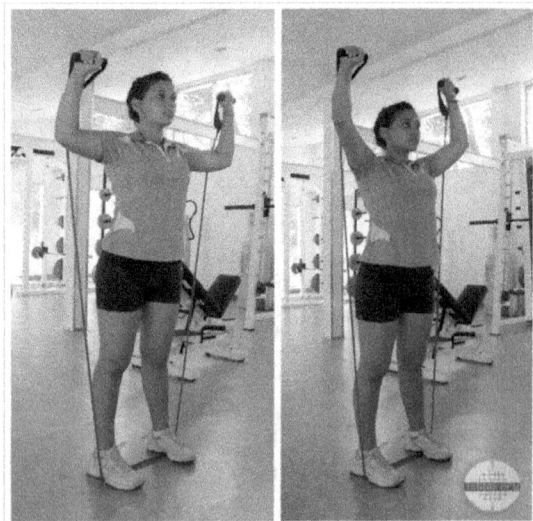

- Start with your palms at shoulder level, facing outward.
- As you contract your shoulders, press the band upward.
- Return to the starting position and repeat.

3) Band Internal Rotation

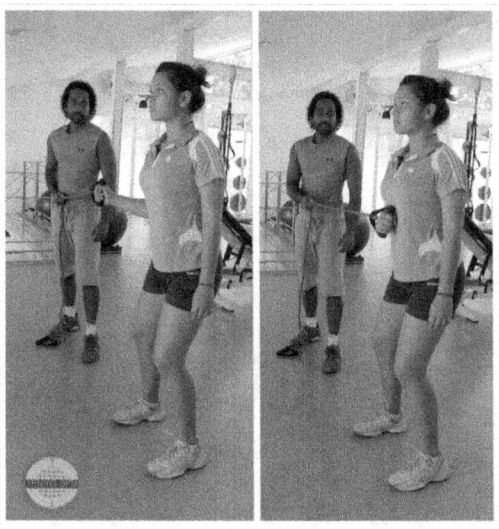

- Hold one arm at a 90-degree angle from your side.
- Pull the band across your midsection to activate your internal rotators.
- Slowly return to the starting position.
- Repeat on both sides.

4) Band External Rotation

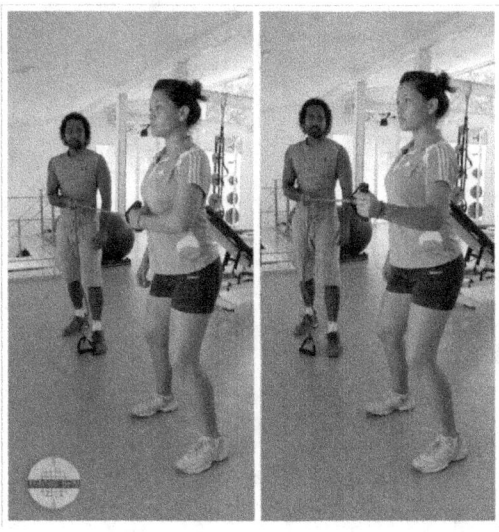

- Start with one arm crossing your midsection as shown in photo 1.
- As you activate the external rotator, pull the band until your arm comes to a 90-degree angle.
- As you progress, you can go beyond this range under supervision, but beginners should stay in the 90-degree range.
- Come back to the starting position and repeat.

5) Dumbbell Front Shoulder Press

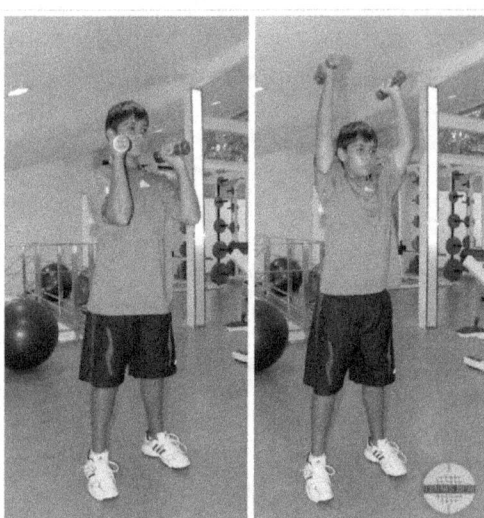

- Start with elbows facing forward and wrists at shoulder level.
- Lift the weights upward as shown in photo 2.
- Return to the starting position and repeat.

6) Dumbbell Side Press

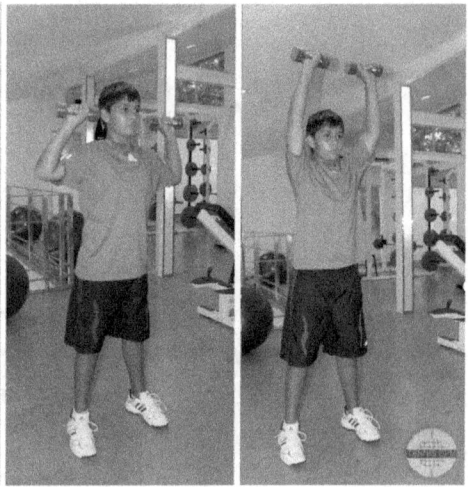

- Start with your elbows raised to almost 90 degrees and your palms facing outward, with wrists at shoulder level.
- Press the weight upward as shown in photo 2.
- Return to the starting position and repeat.

7) Dumbbell Straight Shoulder Raise

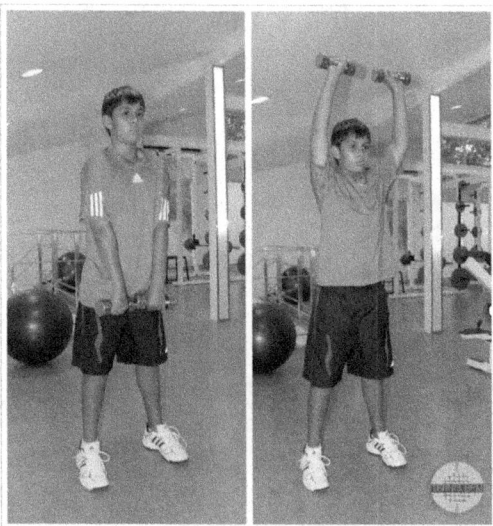

- Start by holding the weights in front of your body with knuckles facing down.
- Keep your arms straight and lift them upward.
- At the end of the motion, your knuckles will point upward as shown in photo 2.
- Return to the starting position and repeat.

8) Dumbbell Lateral Raise

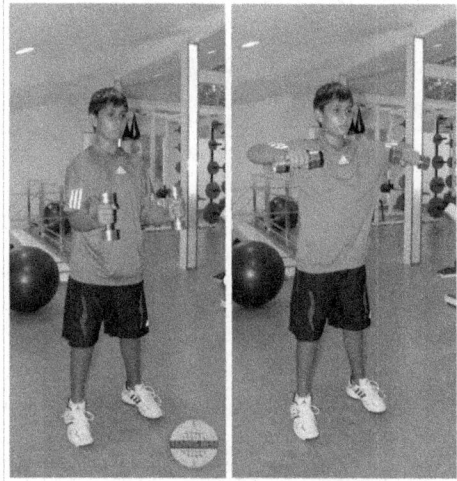

- Start with elbows at 90 degrees with knuckles facing straight ahead vertically as in photo 1.
- By contracting your lateral shoulder muscle, lift your arm so that it's horizontal and knuckles are horizontal as shown in photo 2.
- Return to the starting position and repeat.

9) Dumbbell Internal and External Rotation

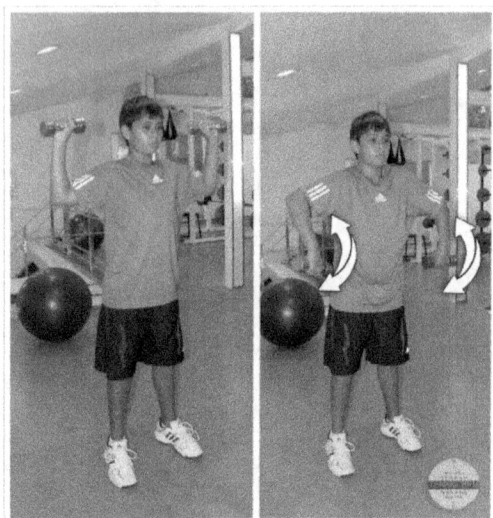

- Start with your elbows at shoulder level at a 90-degree angle and your wrists at the level of your head.
- Lower the weights in a downward movement as shown with arrows. This will activate the internal rotators. From the downward position (as shown in photo 2) follow the arrows up to activate the external rotators.

Abdominals

1) Band Crunch and Twist

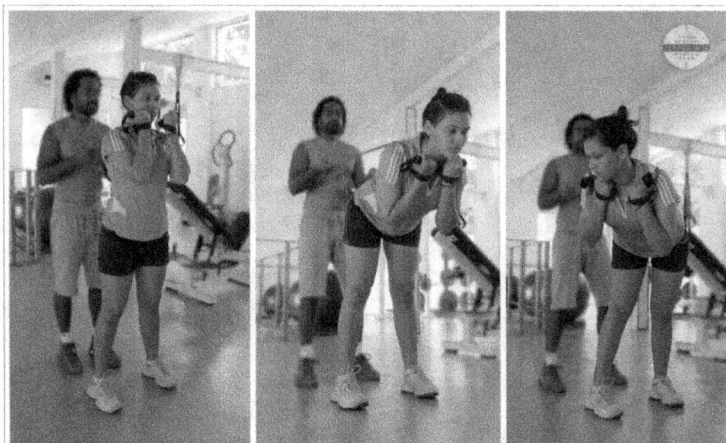

- As shown in photo 1, hold your palms facing your shoulders and step forward until you feel the tension in the band.
- As you contract your abdominals, reach forward and move to the position shown in photo 2, and then return to the starting position.
- As you crunch, twist to the right side as shown in photo 3, return to the starting position, and then crunch and twist to the left side.
- Repeat the exercise.

2) Band Ab Rotation

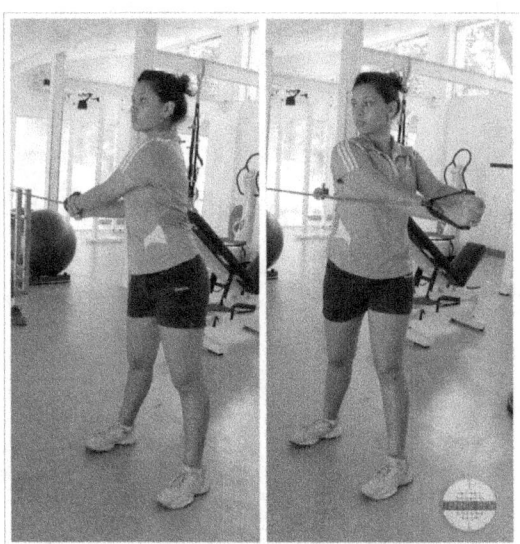

- Start with the band aligned with your right hip as shown in photo 1.
- Keep your fingers interlaced and bring the band across your midsection, contracting your abdominals until the band reaches your left side.
- Return to the starting position and repeat.
- When you complete your target sets and reps, repeat on the other side.

3) Ab Crunch

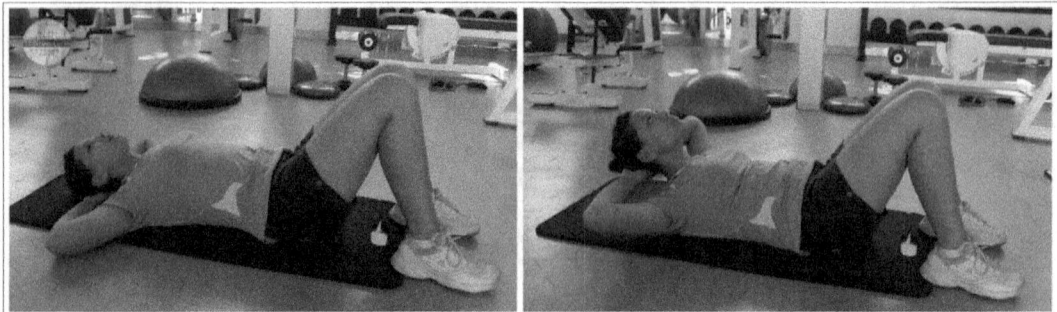

- Keep your lower back flat on the mat and your feet close to your buttocks.
- Lift your shoulder blades off the mat as you contract your abdominals.
- Make sure your chin is facing the ceiling.
- Return to the starting position and repeat.

4) Ab Reverse Crunch

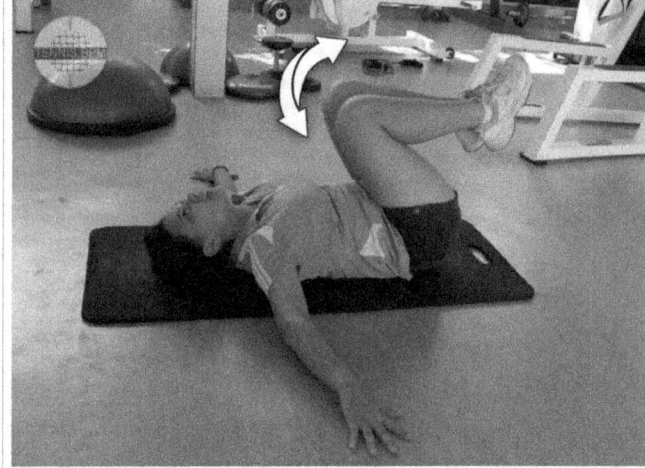

- The photo shows the end motion of this exercise. Your buttocks are slightly raised from the mat and your knees should be in line with your chest.
- Return to the starting position, as demonstrated by the arrows, and repeat.

5) Ab Side Crunch

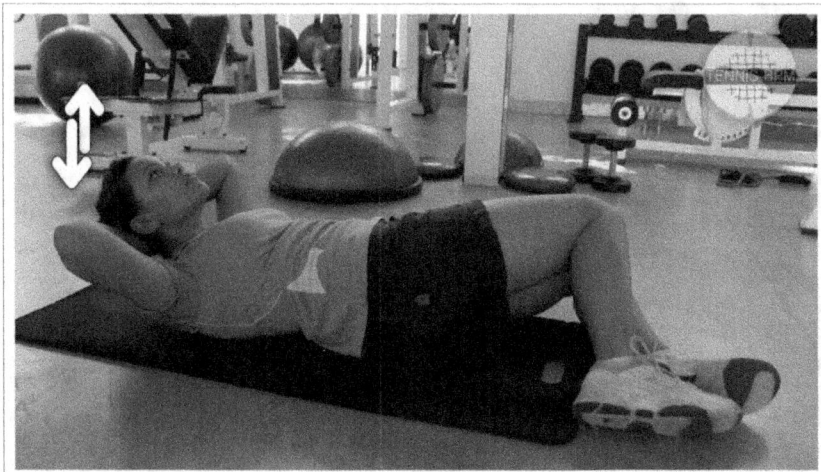

- Start in the same position as for the ab crunch.
- By keeping your knees to the side, you will focus on the side abdominal. This is the only difference from the basic ab crunch.
- From a downward position, move upward as you contract the abs and then return to the starting position. After you complete your sets and reps, repeat the exercise with your knees to the opposite side.

6) Ball Ab Tucks

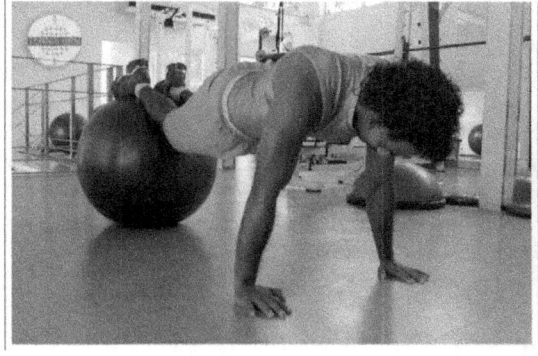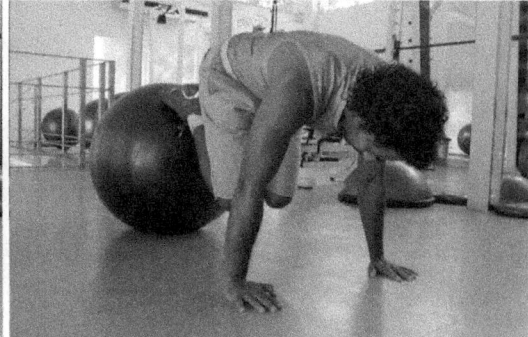

- This is a level-one advanced exercise with many progressions.
- Rest your feet or shins on the ball and place your palms in line with your shoulders. Keep your body as straight as possible.
- As you pull your knees toward your chest, contract your abdominal muscles.
- For variety, you can pull your knees toward your elbows at either side.
- Return to the starting position and repeat.

7) Medicine Ball Rotational Ab Throw (Power)

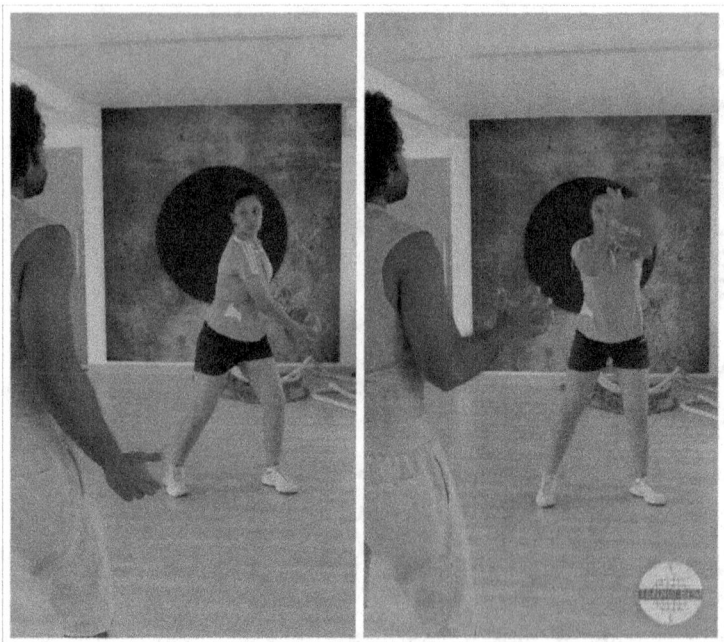

- Start by holding the medicine ball below your hips as shown in photo 1.
- Contract your abdominal muscles as you throw the ball to your partner.
- Return to the starting position and repeat on both sides.

Lower Back

1) **Band Back Reach**

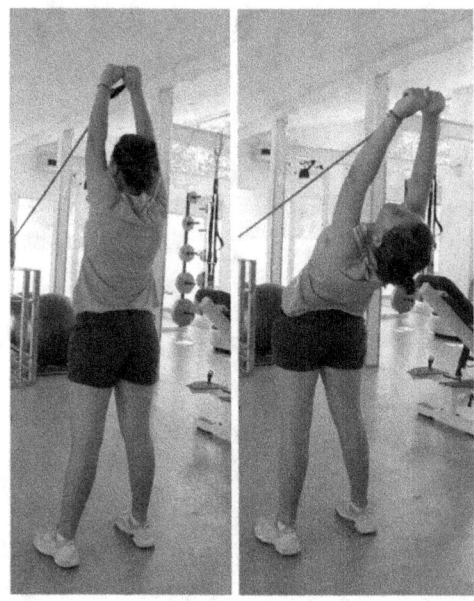

- Stand with arms over your head, holding the band.
- Maintaining this position, flex and contract your lower back muscles, stretching as shown in photo 2.
- Return to the starting position and repeat.

2) Floor Quad Lift

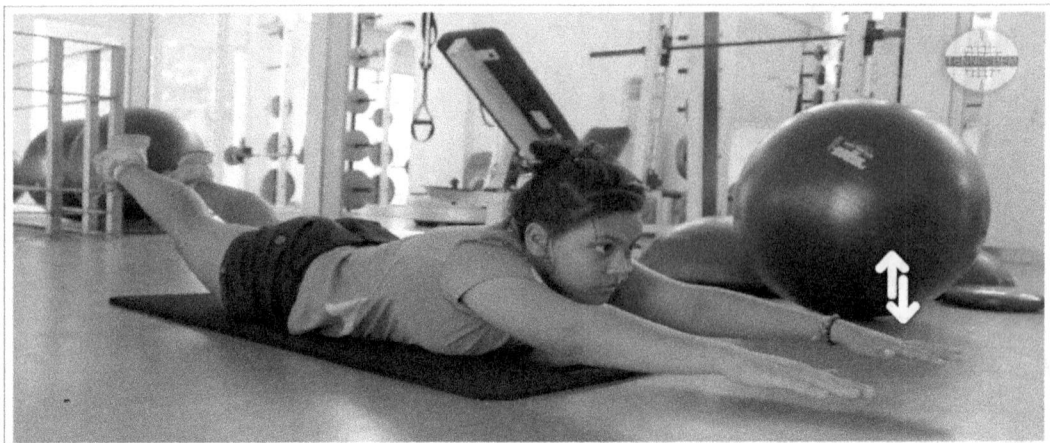

- Start with your arms and legs resting on the floor.
- As you contract your lower-back and buttocks muscles, raise your arms and legs.
- Return to the starting position and repeat, following the arrows in the photo.
- Repeat the exercise.

3) Ball Extension

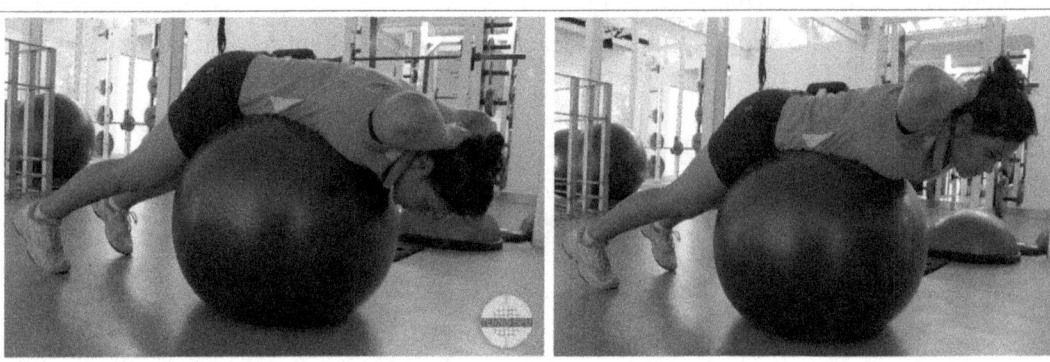

- Start by leaning forward as shown in photo 1.
- Contract your lower back muscles and bring your body into a straight line with your lower back as shown in photo 2.
- Return to the starting position and repeat.

4) Ball Reverse Extension

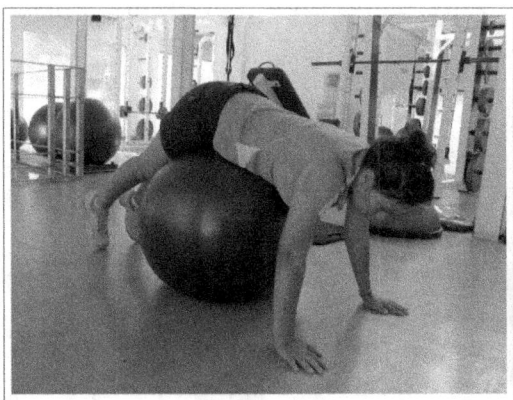 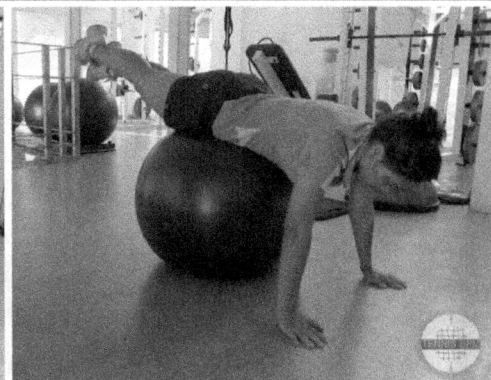

- Start with your stomach resting on the stability ball and your arms and legs resting on the floor.
- As you contract your lower-back muscles and buttocks, lift your legs until they are aligned with your back in a straight line.

5) Medicine Ball Reverse Throw (Power)

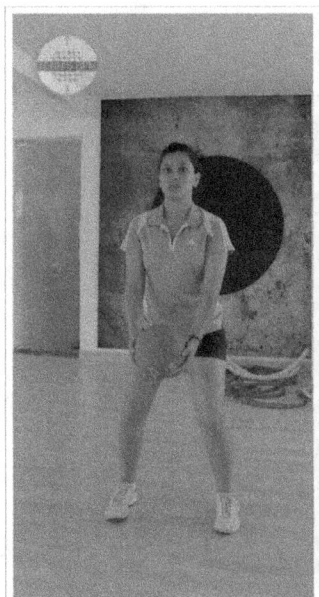 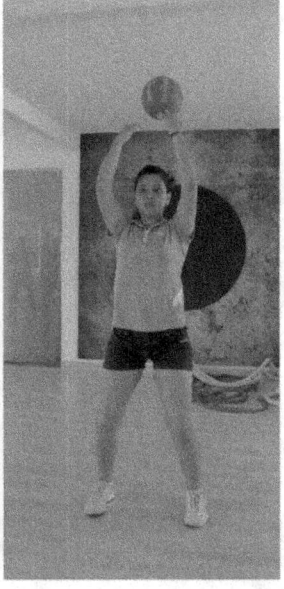

- Stand with your knees slightly bent, holding the medicine ball in front and leaning your upper body forward. As you progress, you can increase the angle at which you lean forward.
- Then use the contraction of your lower-back muscles to throw the ball overhead as shown in photo 2.
- Repeat the exercise.

6) Total Body Medicine Ball Exercise

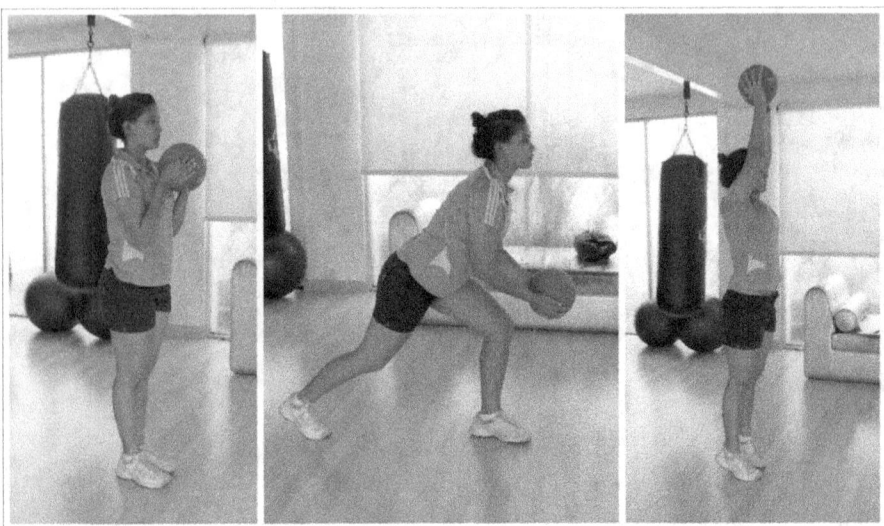

- Start with your feet together, holding the medicine ball close to your chest as shown photo 1.
- Lunge forward with your left leg, and then bring your back leg toward your left leg.
- Curl and press the ball upward as you raise your heels.
- You can repeat this on a single leg or alternate legs each time.

7) Medicine Ball Lunge Rotation

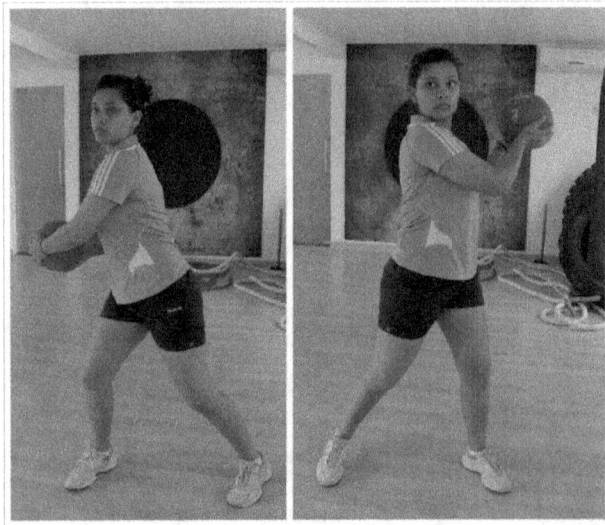

- Slightly bend your right knee and hold the ball by your right hip.
- As you pivot, contract the muscles in your entire body and take the ball up and across your body to your left shoulder.
- Repeat on both sides.

SECTION 6 — SPEED AND AGILITY

Speed

In any sport you play and in daily life, you will come across situations that require sudden speed with or without prior notice. In sports, speed is king. It is produced through a combination of reaction speed, acceleration, endurance speed, and explosive speed. It can also be described as the time taken to coordinate individual joints or the whole body as fast as possible.

The best definition of speed I've seen is: "An individual's ability to execute motor action that cause the body or parts of the body to move quick as possible for short periods of time in absence of fatigue" *(Pradet 1996)*.

Speed strength: Force developed quickly is the foundation of speed training.

Speed endurance: Supports speed and agility over a period of time.

To improve speed, use the methods described below after attaining a solid base of other fitness components, such as stability, flexibility, strength, and power.

a) **Assisted Speed Training**
   - A person is accelerated to a new level that he or she is not comfortable with yet to increase stride frequency (not for beginners).
   - It may or may not benefit movements for tennis. There is no solid evidence proving this; however, it would make sense to train a downhill runner or trekker with assisted speed training rather than tennis players.

b) **Resisted Speed Training**
   Moving from a horizontal position to a vertical position to increase force production in the drive phase and increase stride length.
   1) Lateral

2) Forward
3) Backward

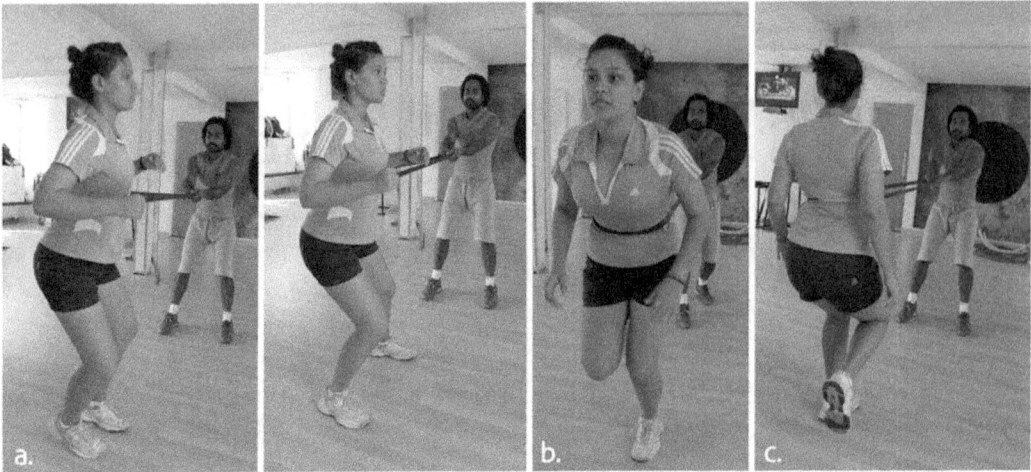

- Photo *a* shows resisted sidestepping from a position with the feet close together. You can open out and repeat the action when you have completed the number of reps and sets. Repeat on the opposite side.
- Photo *b* demonstrates resisted forward running. As your partner holds you back, your aim is to do as many forward runs as possible.
- Photo *c* shows backward running, which follows the same principle as forward running.

Agility

The purpose of agility is to maintain stability (balance) while moving with a combination of multidirectional movements, acceleration, deceleration, stops, and starts.

1) Cone T Drill (Forward, Side, Run, Side, Back)

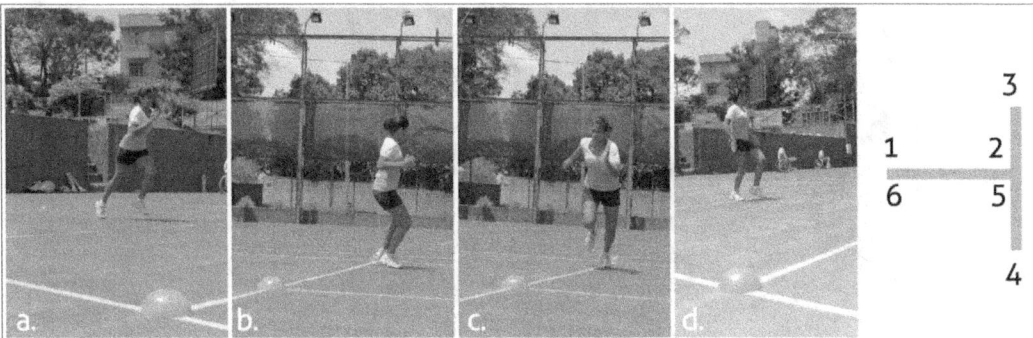

- Set up cone 1 at the center of the baseline, cone 2 at the *T*, cone 3 at the single or doubles line, and cone 4 opposite cone 3.
- Do a forward run to cone 2, as shown in photo *a*.
- From cone 2, do a side step to cone 3 as shown in photo *b*.
- When you reach cone 3, turn around and do a forward run to cone 4, as shown in photo *c*.
  - From cone 4, sidestep to cone 2 (5 in illustration).
- As shown in photo *d*, backward run to starting position 1 (6 in illustration).
- Repeat the same sequence on the opposite side.

2) Forward, Back, Side, and Carioca Drill

I. Agility Carioca

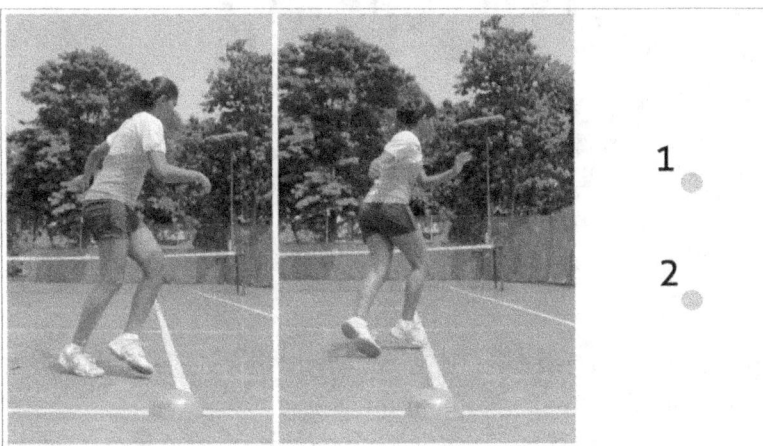

- Place two cones as targets from the baseline to service line.
- Start from cone 2 with your right foot behind your left foot (crossed feet) and then uncross your feet, immediately followed by crossing your right foot in front of the left foot. Repeat between cone 1 and 2 as shown in photo.

II. Cone Forward Run and Backward

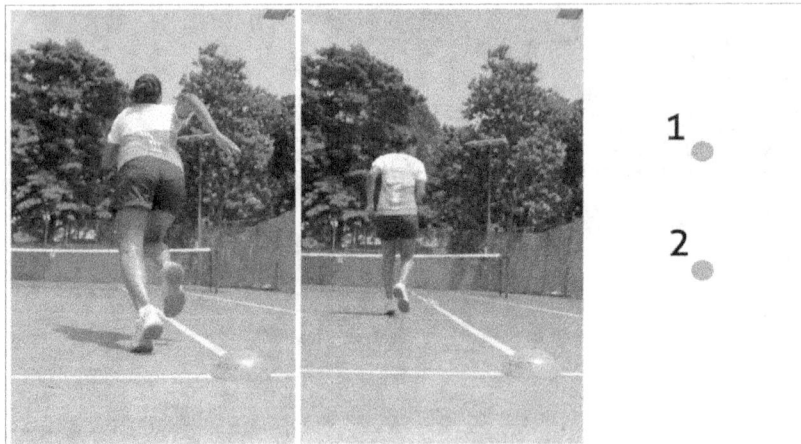

- Run forward from cone 2 to 1, turn around, and do a forward run.
- Then do a backward run as shown in the second photo.
- For agility specific training, you can combine all 4 exercises illustrated in this section.
- Repeat until you complete your reps and sets.

III. Cone Side Step

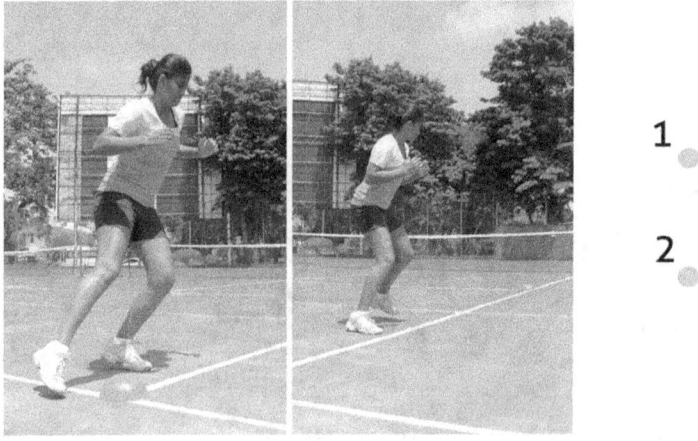

- Step out with your left foot, bring your right foot closer to the left foot, and then step out with the left foot again, forming side steps.
- When you reach a cone, repeat the sequence starting with your right foot.

3) Ladder (Split Step, Side Shuffle, Front Shuffle, Crossover Step, Quick Toe)

I. Ladder Quick Toes

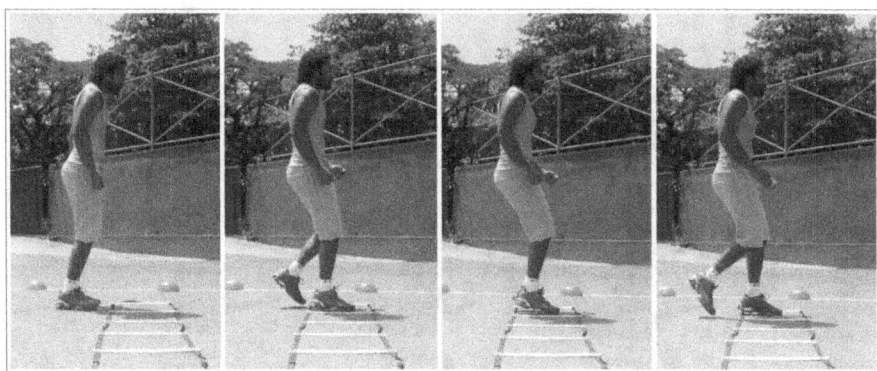

- Face the side of the ladder as shown in photo 1.
- Step into the first ladder box with your right foot as shown in photo 2.
- Quickly bring your left foot to the same box as shown in photo 3.
- Quickly step back with your right foot, followed by the left foot as shown in photo 4.
- Step on the second square with your right foot and repeat the sequence until you reach the end of the ladder.
- After you reach the end, repeat by starting with the left foot till you reach the end.
- Repeat as needed or combine with other drills.

II. Ladder Split

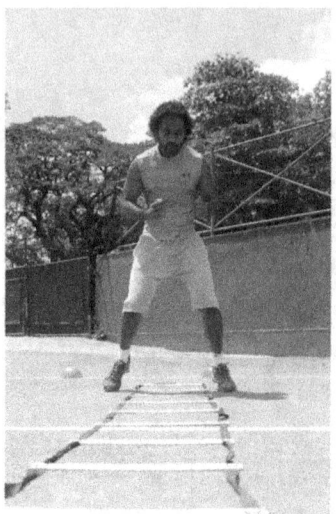

- Start by facing the ladder and placing your feet on each side of the ladder as shown in the photo.
- Keep your heels off the ground and your weight on the balls of your feet.
- Quickly bring both feet inside the ladder box, keeping your heels up.
- Follow this by a split step, also shown in the photo, with feet outside the second box in the ladder. Repeat till you reach the end of the ladder.
- As a variation, you can do a backward split step or turn and repeat the split step forward.

III. Ladder Front Shuffle

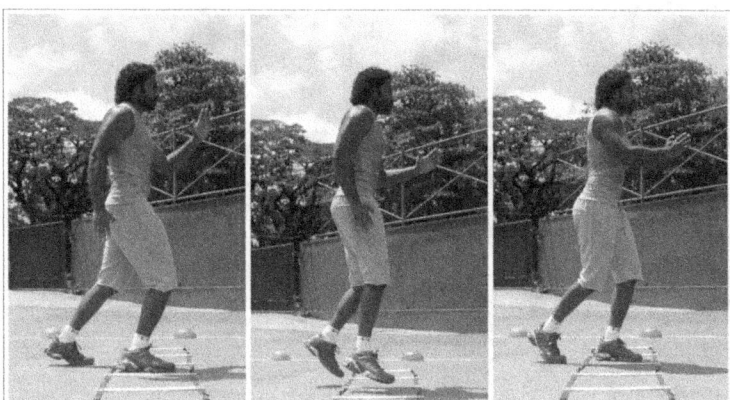

- Use opposite arms and legs, as shown in photo 1. Step forward to put your right leg and left arm in the first box.
- Shuffle feet in the air as shown in photo 2.
- Land with the left leg and right arm in the ladder's second box.
- Repeat the sequence till reaching the end of the ladder.
- Follow the same steps and return to the starting position.

IV. Ladder Side Shuffle

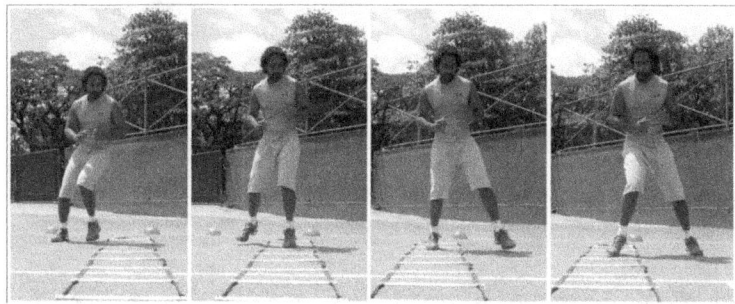

- Start by facing the ladder diagonally by the first box as shown in photo 1.
- Step into the first box with your left foot as shown in photo 2.
- Move your right foot to the first box and your left foot diagonally to the second box as shown in photo 3.
- Bring your right foot next to your left foot.
- Repeat the sequence by diagonally stepping into the second box with your right foot as shown in photo 4.
- Repeat this sequence in a zigzag pattern till you reach the end of the ladder.
- Do the side shuffle backward or turn around and shuffle forward using a similar pattern.

V. Ladder Crossover Step

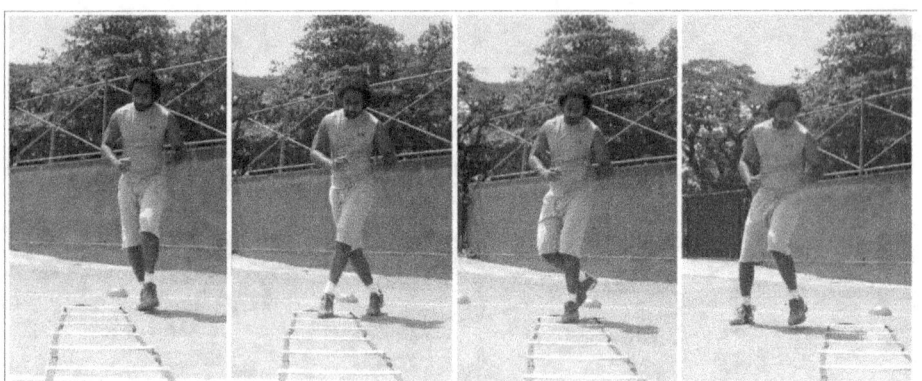

- Start diagonal to the ladder as shown in photo 1.
- Do a crossover step with your left foot and place it in the first box (photo 2).
- Put your right foot in the air as shown in photo 3.
- Place your right foot down, followed by the left foot to end in a diagonal position on the opposite side, as shown in photo 4.
- Repeat the motion with a crossover step from the right foot in the second box.
- Repeat till you reach the end of the ladder.
- You can turn around and repeat this or do a backward crossover step.

SECTION 7 — REACTION AND QUICKNESS

Quickness is doing a particular movement in a short time, called reaction time. When you act on your opponent's movements or other cues, the response time is the reaction time needed to complete the movement. As you can see, speed, agility, quickness, and reaction work together with your mind and direct your body to move through audio or visual cues.

Speed is also main factor in power, as discussed previously.

1) **Reaction Ball Catch and Bounce**

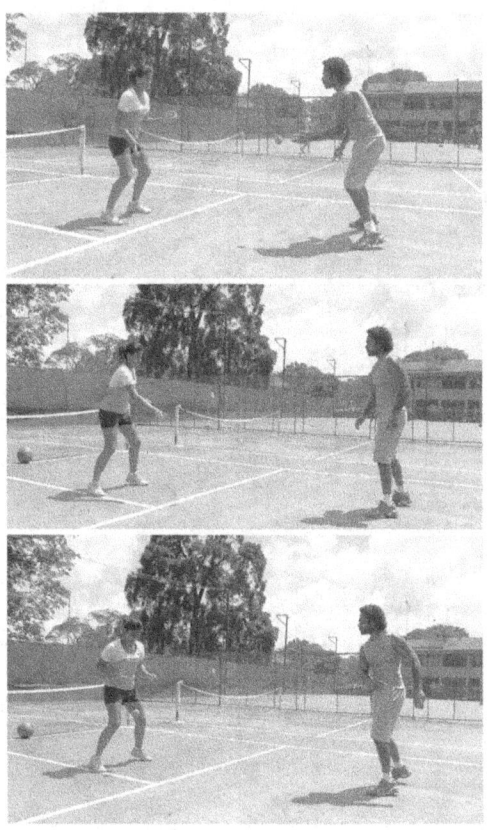

- As shown in the top photo, your partner can throw the ball, and you can respond to the command and catch it.
- Add variety by getting your partner or coach to bounce the ball on the ground as shown in photo 3.
- Another variation could be to catch the ball in a certain number of bounces (e.g., after one or two bounces) or to alternate which hand you catch it with).

2) Ball Drops

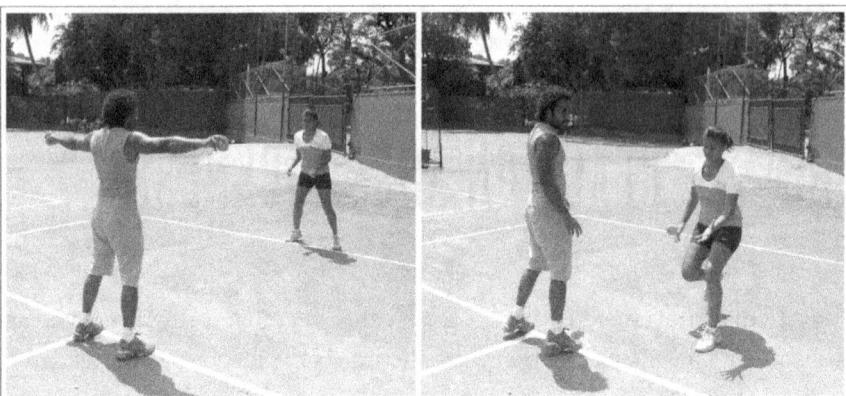

- Your coach or partner stands with his or her arms extended, holding a ball on each side.
- Without warning, that person drops the ball on one side.
- Your goal is to catch it with either your left or right hand. You may alternate sides (e.g., left hand and left foot, right hand and left foot) to create your own combinations.

3) Wall Catches

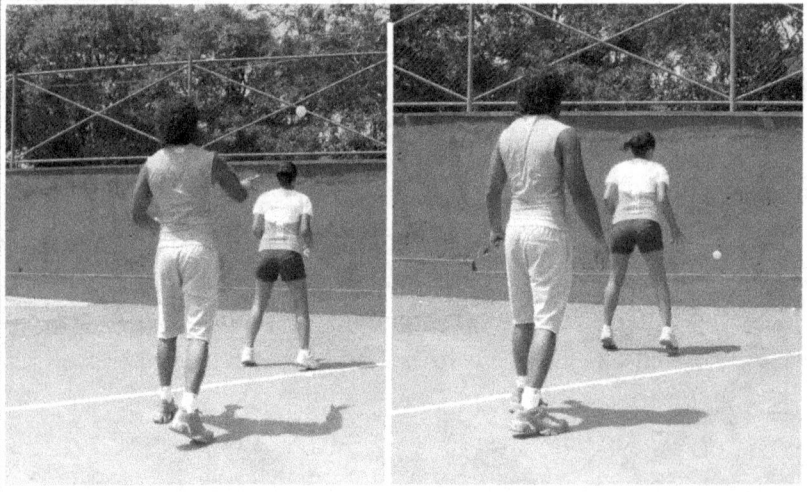

- While you face the wall, your partner or coach will stand behind you, out of visual range.
- Without warning you, he or she throws the ball and calls out a number (e.g., one or two).
- Your goal is to react and catch as many balls as the person announced.
- For variety and increased difficulty, you can catch with either your left or right hand, or alternate sides, or create your own combinations.

4) Copy Partner

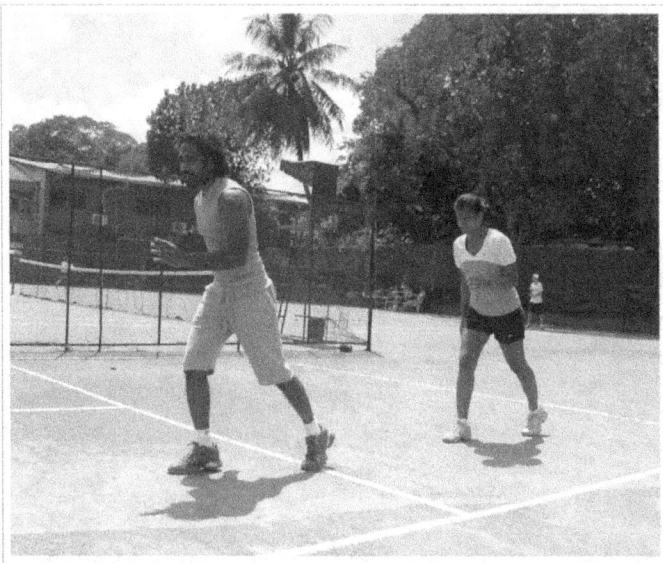

- Stand behind your coach or partner.
- He or she will run in multiple directions with different arm gestures.
- Your goal is to copy each and every movement.

5) Mirror Partner

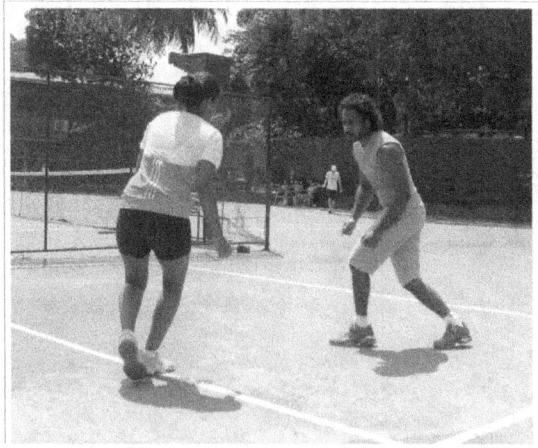

- Start by facing your partner or coach.
- Try to copy every moment, from multidirectional running to hand gestures.
- Keep your eyes focused on him or her.

6) Quick Feet

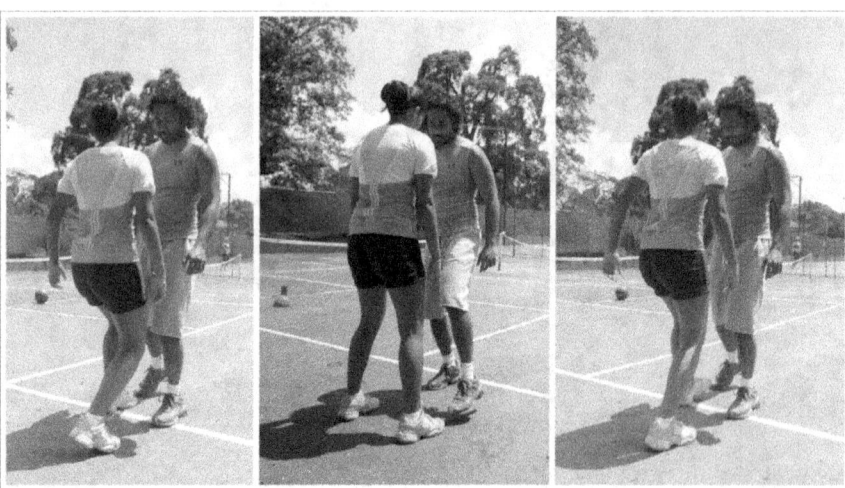

- Start by facing your partner or coach.
- As shown in photo 1, you can try to step on either of his or her feet. If you do, you get a point. If not, return to the starting position as shown in photo 2.
- Without warning you, your partner will try to step on your feet. You need to move your feet before that happens, trying to step on his or her feet.
- Create your own variations.

7) Quick Arms

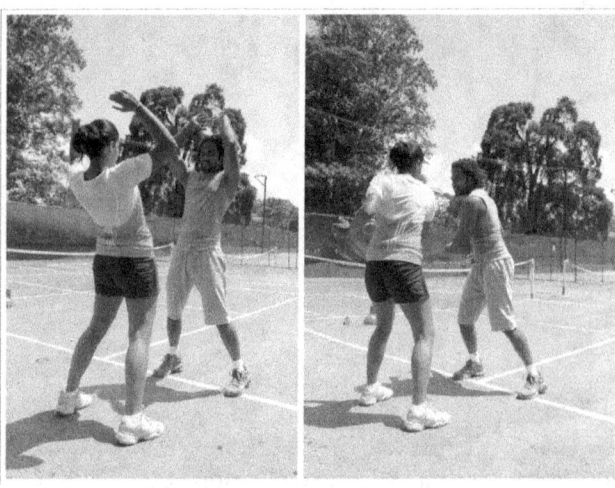

- Start by facing your partner or coach.
- Copy arm movements as shown in photo 1.
- Copy arm and upper-body movements as shown in photo 2.
- Reverse the exercise with your partner or coach.

Plyometrics

Plyometrics is a part of strength training. It's a quick and powerful movement (like a bow and arrow). An eccentric contraction is immediately followed by concentric contraction.

Refer to the upper-body and lower-body power exercises in the strength training section.

SECTION 8 — COOLDOWN AND STATIC FLEXIBILITY

A cooldown is like the opposite of a warm-up. It allows your body to gradually transition from an exertion state to a resting state.

A good indicator of a successful cooldown is a decreasing heart rate. For example, a slow jog or walk removes the production of metabolic waste as a result of exercise.

Static Stretching
Hold the stretch to improve the length of the contracted muscle or group of muscles, thereby improving flexibility.

Duration
Hold the stretch for 30–40 seconds.
Sets: repeat 1–2 times for each muscle or group

1) Back of thighs
2) Front of thighs
3) Buttocks
4) Calves
5) Inner thigh
6) Outer thigh and inner abdominals
7) Chest
8) Upper arms
9) Back of the arms
10) Armpit Stretch
11) Shoulder side

12) Shoulder rotator
13) Mid and upper back
14) Lower back
15) Forearm (front)
16) Forearm (back)
17) Neck

1) Back Thigh Stretch

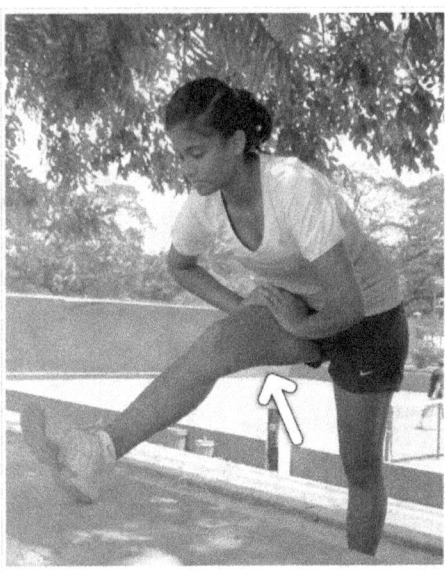

- Keep your right knee slightly bent.
- Place your hands on the top of your right thigh as shown in the photo and bend over from the waist.
- You should feel a slight stretch in your back thigh muscle.
- Repeat on both sides an equal number of times.

2) Front Thigh

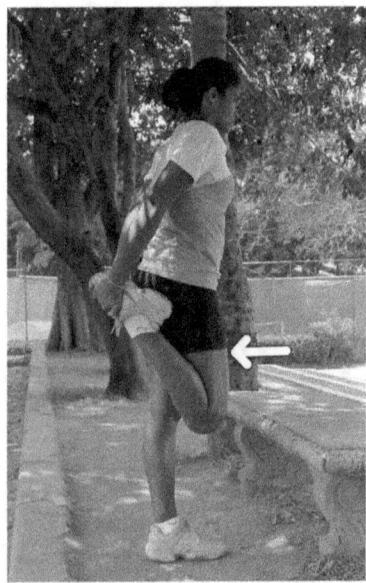

- Keeping your body straight, grab your right foot with your right hand. Repeat with the left.
- Feel the stretch along the front of the thigh, as shown by the arrow in the photo.
- Repeat on both sides.

3) Buttocks

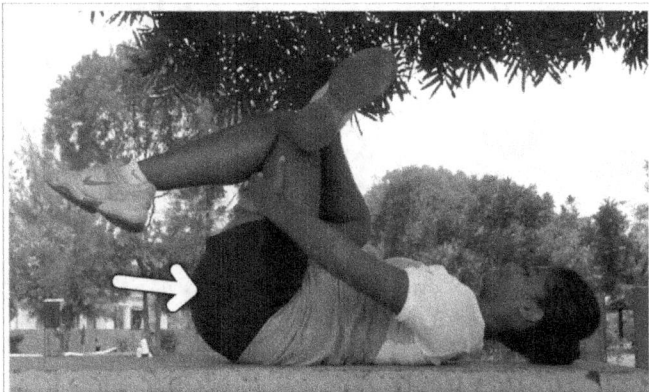

- Life flat on a bench or the floor.
- Place your right ankle on top of your left knee.
- Pull your left thigh toward your body until you feel a slight stretch in your buttock as shown with the arrow.
- Repeat on the opposite side.

4) Calves

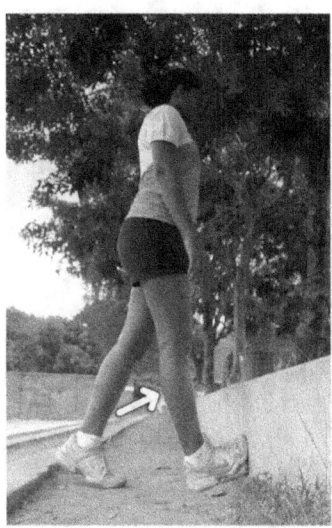

- Keep your body straight and lock your right knee.
- Place your toes against a tree or ledge so they are facing the sky, as shown in the photo.
- Feel the stretch in the calf region as indicated by the arrow.
- Repeat on the other side.

5) Inner Thigh

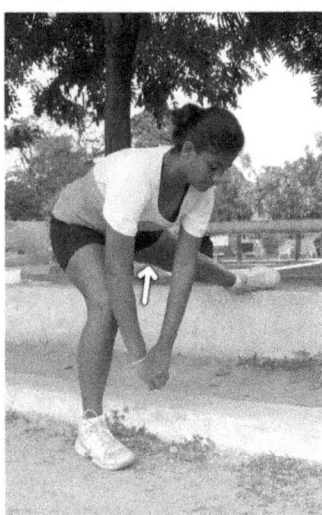

- Put your left foot on a step, bench, or ledge as shown in the photo.
- Transfer your weight slightly onto the right leg while keeping a straight back and leaning forward with your arms.
- This will enable you to feel the stretch in the inner thigh as shown by the arrow.
- Repeat on the opposite side.

6) IT Band and Overall Stretch

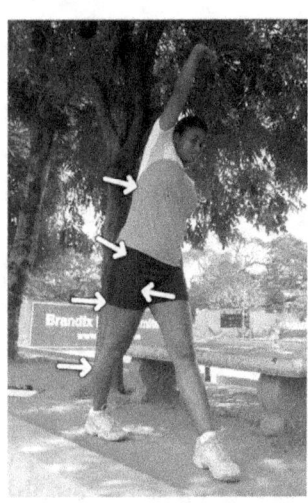

- Place your left foot in front of you, your right foot behind your body, and raise your right hand toward the sky.
- Lock your back knee and slightly lean forward from the right hip.
- Push your right hip out slightly, followed by the right upper body as shown in the photo.
- Starting from the top arrow, this will stretch the entire side of your upper body, followed by inner abdominal region (psoas), the IT (Iliotibial) band side of the thigh, the calves, and finally the upper-thigh region.
- Repeat on the opposite side.

7) Chest Stretch

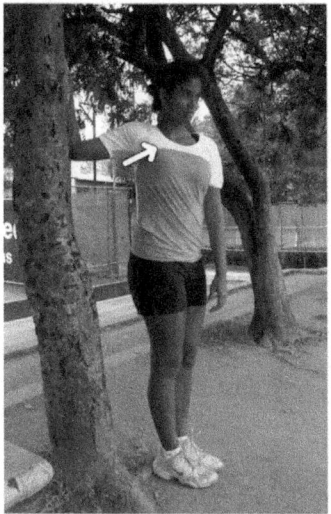

- Stand with your elbow at a 90-degree angle against a tree or wall as shown in the photo.
- Slightly rotate your hips until you feel the stretch in your chest region.
- Repeat on the opposite side.

8) Upper-Arm Stretch

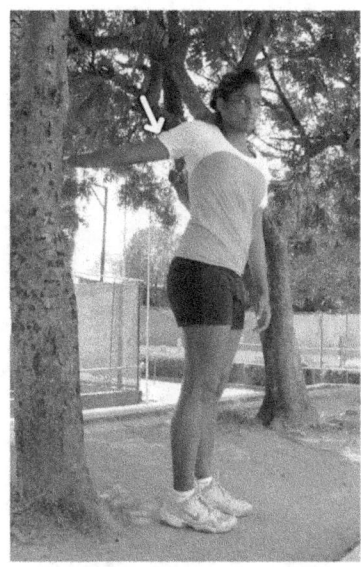

- Clench your right fist and extend the arm against a tree or a wall.
- Slightly rotate your hips until you feel the stretch on your bicep, as shown by the arrow.
- Repeat on the other side.

9) Back of the Arm

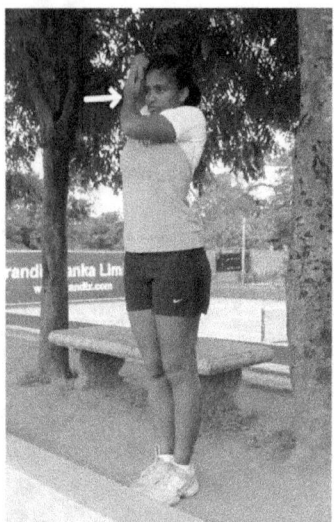

- Stand straight with your right hand bent and right elbow pointing forward as shown in the photo.
- Push your right elbow gently with your left hand so that you feel the stretch where the arrow is pointing.
- Repeat on the opposite side.

10) Armpit Stretch

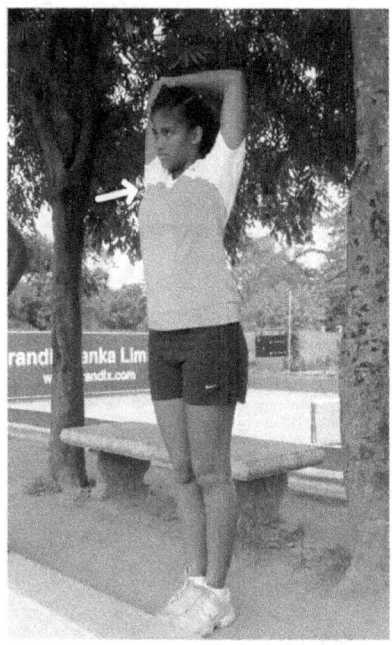

- Stand straight with your right hand bent and your right elbow pointing out to the right side as shown in the photo.
- Push your right elbow gently with your left hand so that you feel the stretch, as shown with the arrow in the photo.
- Repeat on the opposite side.

11) Shoulder Stretch

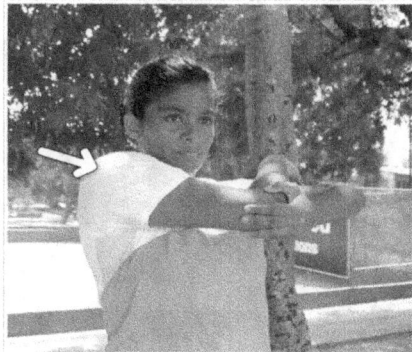

- Stand straight, bend your right elbow, and take your arm across your body as shown in the photo.
- Pull your right elbow gently with your left hand.
- Feel the stretch on the shoulder region as shown by the arrow.

12) Inside Shoulder Stretch

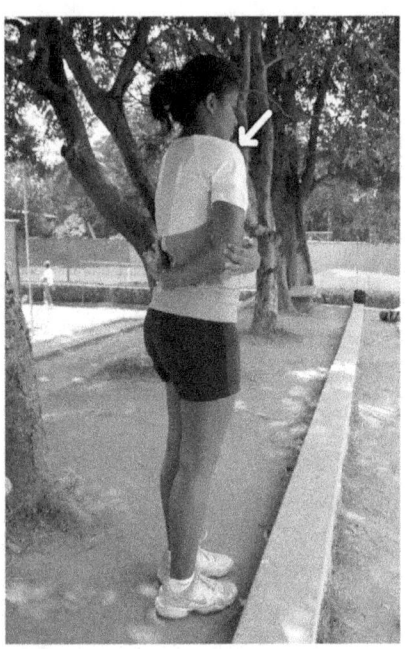

- Stand straight and keep your right hand bent as shown in the photo.
- Make sure your right palm is turned outward.
- Using your left hand, gently pull your right elbow toward the front of your body.
- This will stretch the shoulder region shown by the arrow.
- Repeat on the opposite side.

13) Mid and Upper Back Stretch

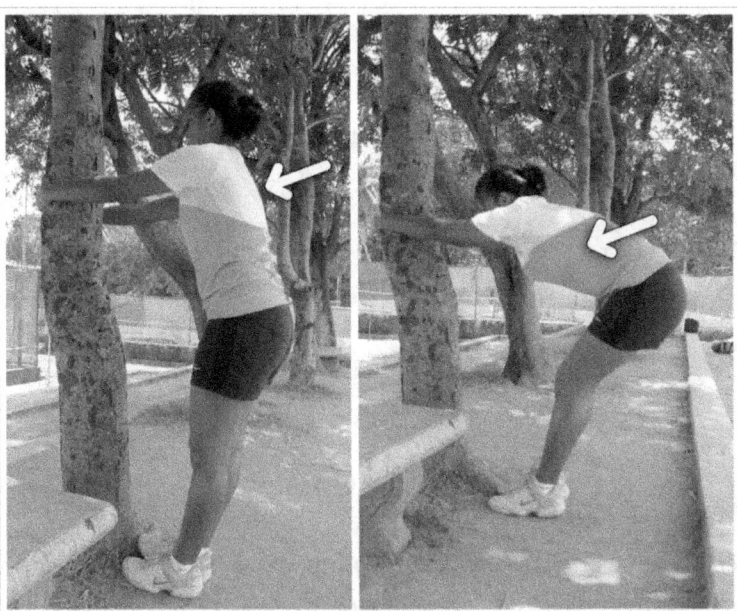

- Grab a tree or pillar for support.
- Curve your upper back muscle and transfer the weight as shown in photo.
- You will feel the stretch in the area shown by the arrow.

14) Lower Back Stretch

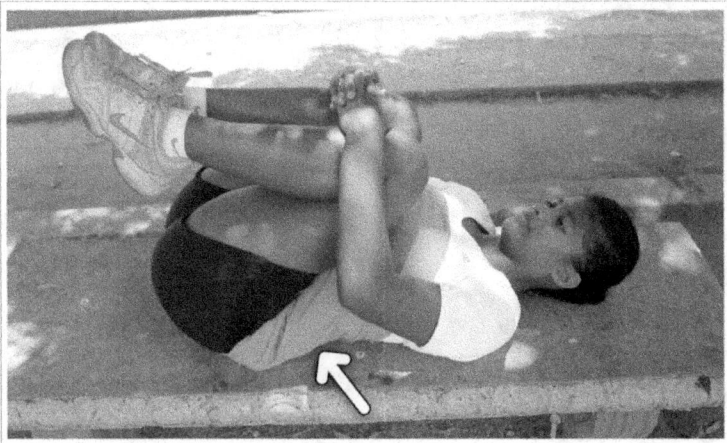

- Lie flat on the floor or bench.
- Wrap your arms around your knees and hug them tightly.
- Try to pull your knees toward your chest.
- Feel the stretch in your lower back as shown by the arrow.

15) Forearm (front)

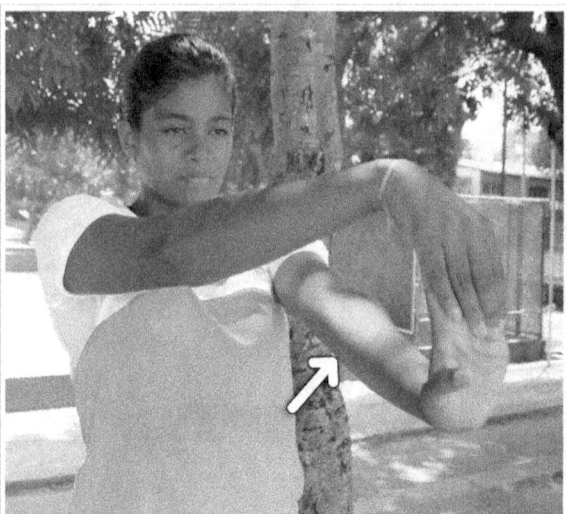

- Stand straight with your left arm extended and fingers pointing up.
- Use your right hand to pull back the fingers of your left hand.
- This will stretch the region of the forearm shown by the arrow.
- Repeat on the opposite side.

16) Forearm (back)

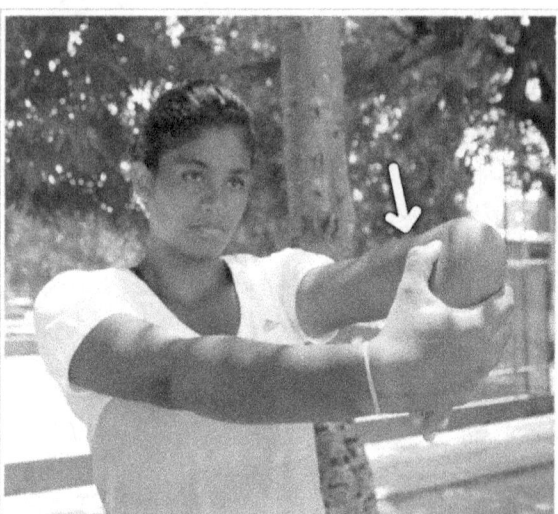

- Stand straight, with your left arm extended and fingers pointing downward.
- Use your right hand to pull the left wrist and fingers toward the body.
- This will stretch the region indicated by the arrow.
- Repeat on the opposite side.

17) Neck Stretch

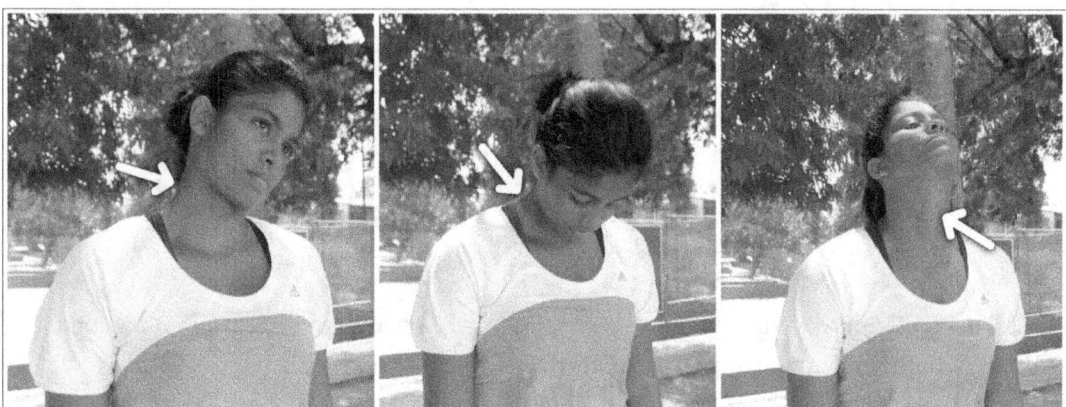

- As shown in photo 1, bend your left ear toward your left shoulder. By doing this motion, you will feel the stretch on the right side of your neck as shown by the arrow.
- As shown in photo 2, bend your chin toward the ground, thereby stretching the back of the neck as shown by the arrow.
- Finally, raise your chin toward the sky, enabling you to feel the stretch in the front of your neck as shown in photo 3.

SECTION 9 — NUTRITION

Note: This section is for informational purposes only. Consult your medical professional and registered dietitian before using these or any other dietary guidelines.

Hydration

According to research, sustaining a fluid loss of even 1% of your body weight has negative effects to:
a) Physical fitness
b) Blood volume
c) Electrolytes
d) Muscle contraction

This is because sweat reduces body heat, and water absorbs heat from the muscles to reduce the temperature. Approximately 90 percent of your blood is used to transport nutrients to working muscles and to get rid of byproducts. Saliva and gastrointestinal secretions help to digest the food and turn it into liquid. The key factors to consider are the activities you do and the weather conditions.

The best way to check whether you are dehydrated is to check your urine in the morning (the darker the urine, the more waste products it contains). If it is close to clear or the color of lemonade, it is a good indicator that you are properly hydrated.

If you are well-hydrated, the way to assess your water loss is to check your weight on a scale before and after any exercise or sport activity you are planning to do. The weight immediately after the activity shows loss of water.

According to leading fitness, exercise and strength and conditioning organizations, the amount of recommended hydration for activity can be summarized as seen below.

Before activity: drink 14–20 oz. two hours before activity.

During activity: drink 6–12 oz. sports drink every fifteen to twenty minutes of sweaty exercise.

After activity: drink 16–24 oz. water and sports drink to replace the pounds that you lost.

Hydration helps prepare you for the task at hand, gives you energy during the activity, and acts as recovery agent afterward.

Dehydration
If you are feeling thirsty, you are dehydrated. This is caused by the temperature, humidity, pre-hydration status, improper clothing or insufficient acclimatization.

Signs of Dehydration

Stage 1
Thirst, flushed skin, muscle cramps

Stage 2
Dizziness, vomiting, nausea, chills, shortness of breath

It's best to address the issue before you notice symptoms of stage two.

Rehydration
A sports drink should contain less than 8% carbohydrates and around 6% sodium.

To replace your water and electrolyte loss, Mix the following ingredients to make an easy homemade sports drink.

200–250 ml fruit juice (ideally Orange)
800 ml water
1g salt

Why Nutrition Is Key

This is the area most people are misled. Women search for the next quick-fix diet to lose fat and weight, men seek to have a ripped, muscular body, and athletes try to find the super supplement so that they can have a competitive edge by improving their size, speed, power, endurance etc.

The human body is meant to function in a specific way. Some of the primary reasons we need nutrition are:

    a.   To maintain and repair the body's cells and tissue
    b.   To provide energy to survive
    c.   To provide energy for sports and other recreational activities
    d.   For growth (kids and teens)

Imagine that you drive a sports car. Could you operate it without gas, engine oil, water, power, steering fluid, brake fluid or a battery? This analogy applies to your body, as it needs carbohydrates, protein, fat, vitamins, and minerals to perform optimally.

If you are an average person with a day job, your need for food is different from an athletic person or a model. Your registered dietitian can assess you and recommend a meal plan accordingly.

The scope of this section is to simplify and help you understand more about nutrition without bombarding you with words you cannot understand and tricky marketing names that make you think you are eating healthy when something is really processed food with artificial colors.

I tell all my clients as a rule of thumb, "If it comes in box or bottle with unreadable ingredients, stay clear of it." Natural food such as fruits, vegetables, fish, meats, and milk do not have a long expiration date. If you have food with a longer expiration date, it is usually packed with preservatives, additives, and other chemicals to increase the shelf life.

Food can be broken down into the following categories.

1) **Want Food**—What you like or crave based on its look, smell, and taste (it's usually high in sugar or fat and processed). These foods have a negative impact on health and performance and can lead to the onset of many diseases.

2) **Need Food**—What your body needs to function. These are usually natural whole foods, such as meats, fish, vegetables, fruits, and water that have positive effects on health and performance and offer disease prevention.

Need Food

Raw, Unprocessed and Organic
The current trend is to eat raw and organic food, but what does this mean? Organic foods are free of chemicals or they are grown in a place free of fertilizer and pesticides. Chances are that the chemicals from inorganic food will eventually affect our bodies in a negative way.

If you have access to organic and raw food, by all means, go for it. They preserve the enzymes which help digestion by supplying energy and maintaining metabolism, as stewing, micro-waving, freezing, blackening, and grilling kills certain enzymes and vitamins. This is a better option than processed food, so that you can have a peace of mind that it is chemical-free.

Carbohydrates

Good carbohydrates are fruits, whole bread, vegetables, and anything complete with natural sugars. They maintain the natural nutrients when compared with simple sugars and refined carbohydrates that will fluctuate your blood sugar levels. With added sugar cravings, eventually these carbohydrates will be stored as fats. For further understanding, let's get into some of the details.

Carbohydrates are the like gasoline in our bodies. This is the fuel you burn when you exercise, especially above 65% of your VO2 max; refer to the cardiovascular section.

Carbohydrates are stored in the muscle and liver as glycogen and in the blood as glucose.

An average requirement of carbohydrates per day is about four to five grams per lean kilogram of body weight. A gram of carbohydrates produces four calories of energy. There are three main categories of carbohydrates.

Monosaccharides
a. *Glucose or blood sugar*
   This is the primary energy substitute for cells. Also composed of glycogen (muscle and liver); in a sports drink, this appears as dextrose.
b. *Fructose*
   This is naturally produced in fruits and vegetables and used in carbonated drinks. This can decrease insulin; therefore, too much fructose can cause gas and diarrhea.
c. *Galactose*
   Milk sugar

Disaccharides
a. Sucrose from fruits, table sugar (glucose and fructose), and brown sugar.
b. Lactose (glucose and galactose) in Mammalian milk or maltose (glycogen and glucose). Occurs when polysaccharides are broken down for digestion.
c. Fermentation in alcohol (primarily carbs in beers)

Polysaccharides
a. Complex carbohydrates (starch, fiber, glycogen)
b. Starch—plant glucose (greens, nuts, legumes, vegetables)
c. Fiber—plant cell wall formation of carbs (cellulose, hemicellulose, beta-glycogen, pectin)

Fiber resists being broken down in the human digestion system and increase the bulk and water content and decrease the time for feces.
The liver has high glycogen levels; glucogenisis is the process of converting many end products of digestion to glycogen. Glycogen is formed of animal tissue.

What Is the Glycemic Index? (GI Index)

This index groups food by how high and how long it takes to reach an increased blood glucose level.

High GI: increases blood glucose and insulin

Low GI: slower and gradual increase in blood glucose

A) **GI 90–100**
Examples: waffles, donuts, bagels, cornflakes, glucose, pineapple, raisins, carrots, baked potato, watermelon, bread.

B) **GI 60–90**
Examples: Lactose, muffins, all-bran cereal, oat bran, white rice, brown rice, ice cream (low fat), bananas, canned fruit, grapes, oranges, peas, baked beans, pears, sweet potatoes, oatmeal cookies, chocolate, popcorn, potato chips.

C) **GI below 60**
Examples: Barley, rye, milk, yogurt, apples, cherries, grapefruit, plums, chickpeas, kidney beans, lentils, pinto beans, tomatoes, peanuts.

Note: Low levels of fiber in your diet can be associated with constipation, heart problems, colon cancer, diabetes, and other conditions.

A minimum of fifty grams of good sources of fiber (fruits, vegetables, nuts, seeds, legumes) is recommended.

Protein

Amino acids are molecules that join together to form protein.

Out of twenty amino acids, there are twelve nonessential types (can be synthesized in the body) and nine essential varieties (can't be produced in the body and must be ingested as food).

Proteins are essential for recovery and growth of skeletal muscle, organs, and bone tissue. It functions to transport enzymes, antibodies, lipoproteins, hormones, hemoglobin, and albumin in the body.

Positive Proteins

Vegetable proteins are easy for the body to break down and digest. However, if you are an athlete or a highly active person, you might need animal proteins such as those found in fish, white meat, and red meat to get the full spectrum of amino acids (protein compounds). It is alright to have plant-based protein, but consult with a registered dietitian for recommended amounts.

Negative Proteins

Some red meat can be acidic, which makes it difficult to digest because of a high fat content. This type of meat is also associated with diseases, including heart and colon cancer.

Even cow's milk can be hard to digest for many due to the fat content or lactose intolerance. Soy milk and rice milk are good alternatives.

Why Protein Is Your Repair Tool

1. Aids growth and maintains tissue
2. Synthesizes enzymes and hormones
3. Builds antibodies
4. Maintains balance for fluids and electrolytes
5. Repairs muscle damage
6. Provides energy: four calories come from one gram of protein
7. Sustains blood glucose when glycogen drops via gluconeogenesis

Athletes and kids might need extra protein due to their levels of activity, growth, and recovery. The amount of calories someone takes in should not outdo the number of calories he or she burns. Your intake of calories should be adjusted to ensure protein is not your only energy source.

Below is a guideline of protein intake per each kilogram of lean body weight:

Average person: 0.8–0.9g per kg
Endurance athlete: 1.2g per kg
Strength athlete: 1.6–1.8g per kg

The quality of a type of protein can be rated by whether a protein supplies the necessary amino acids proportional to a body's requirements.

a) High-quality animal protein: eggs, meat, fish, poultry, and dairy

b) Low-quality protein (contain few essential amino acids): grains, beans, and vegetables (soy protein is a better option)

By consuming excess protein it will not give you any added benefits as excess proteins are broken down, and the nitrogen excretes as urea in urine. Remaining are used for energy through being converted to carbohydrates (gluconeogenesis) or stored as body fat.

a) Whey Protein (as in cow's milk-cheese) has the highest biological value of any protein by quickly releasing amino acids to the blood stream. Due to this reason it has become a favorite amongst the fitness and sports communities.

b) Casein, is 80 % of the protein in milk and cheese, moderates and prolongs the release of amino acids. It is a slow releasing protein compared with whey protein, nonetheless, it has proven to be beneficial as a complete protein.

c) Egg: This is another slow releasing complete protein with full spectrum of amino acids which is affordable and well tolerated for digestion even for people with milk intolerance.

Fat and Lipids
The word "fat" has a bad reputation, as everyone has been preconditioned to think like that. However, fat is good, provided you select the right types; some are essential to your body.

Healthy Fats

Nuts, seeds, fish, and avocados are good fats that help the metabolism. That's why they are called EFA (essential fatty acids). As your body can't produce them, you need to take them externally in foods like fish (tuna, salmon, or mackerel), flaxseed, and sunflower seeds.

Negative Fats

These are substances that will block your arteries, usually found in red meat, butter, pastries etc. and they will increase your cholesterol. As your body can't process saturated fats, it will store them as blood fat and adipose tissue (fat between your skin and muscles).

Hydrogenated fat (a process that hardens vegetable oils) is found in margarine, sweets, and ice cream. Hydrogenated fat can be more harmful than trans fat, as it has a direct link to heart disease, cancer, and diabetes. It interferes with the metabolism's breakdown of EFAs, increases bad cholesterol (LDL), and decreases good cholesterol (HDL).

Chemically fats consist of carbon, oxygen, and hydrogen. Because fatty acids have more carbon than protein or carbohydrates, they provide nine calories per gram.

Triglycerides (found in fats and oils) are composed of fatty compounds such as sterol, phospholipids, cholesterol, and other common lipids in food.

How much fat is stored in a person's body is related in part to saturated fatty acids (amount of hydrogen content).

a. Saturated fatty acids; will increase bad cholesterol –LDL
    Coconut, palm or animal-based oil

b. Unsaturated fatty acids; will increase good cholesterol HDL

    Monounsaturated: olive, peanut or canola oil.
    Polyunsaturated: soy, corn, sunflower or safflower oil.

Benefits of Fat
1. Stores energy, primarily in adipose tissue.
2. Insulates and protects organs.
3. Facilitates hormone regulation.

4. Carries fat-soluble vitamins A, D, E, and K and essential fatty acids; linoleic acid (omega- 6), and lenolenic acid (omega-3).
5. Vital for formation of cell membranes, function of nervous system, and production of hormones.
6. Provides taste and feeling of satiety after meals.
7. Assists with smooth muscle contraction.

Benefits of Cholesterol
1. Important for structural and functional components of cell membranes.
2. Necessary for production of bile salt, vitamin D, and several sex hormones.
3. Synthesizes cortisol in liver and intestines.

Keep in mind that reducing fat to an extreme level could cause deficiencies in proteins, calcium, iron, and zinc.

When to Reduce Fat
1. If you need to increase carbs in your diet for performance.
2. For total calorie reduction in weight loss.
3. To decrease blood cholesterol.

It is recommended by leading health and fitness organizations that 30% of a person's calories come from fat: 20% from mono- and polyunsaturated fat and 10% from saturated fat. If less than 15% of your diet includes fat, your levels of testosterone, metabolism, muscle development, antioxidants, vitamins, and minerals will drop.

Antioxidants are micronutrients used in metabolism to facilitate immunity and protect your body from oxidative stress (e.g., vitamins A, C, E, and selenium). They balance oxidative stress created by free radicals, as it increases with exercise, work stress, emotional stress.

Vitamins
These organic substances perform certain metabolic functions within your body.

1. Vitamin A: Repairs body tissue, skin, and vision
   Food sources: liver, milk, egg yolks

2. Beta-carotene: Antioxidant
   Food sources: carrots, sweet potatoes, yams, spinach, kale, turnip, papayas, asparagus

3. Calciferol (Vitamin D): Absorbs calcium, increases bone mass, and prevents bone loss.
    Food sources: fish, salmon, oyster, tuna, fortified cereal, milk, wheat germ.

4. Tocopherol (Vitamin E): Antioxidant, aids growth and development
    Food sources: vegetable oil, almonds, pistachios, peanut butter.

5. Phyllorunione (Vitamin K): Blood clotting and bone health
    Food sources: kale, brussels sprouts, spinach, broccoli, avocados, bell peppers, strawberries, cauliflower, tomatoes

6. Ascorbic Acid (Vitamin C): Cell development, healing, and antioxidant; makes iron available for hemoglobin production
    Food sources: sweet peppers, oranges, limes, raspberries, onions, cantaloupe, tomato, grapefruit.

7. Thiamin (Vitamin B1): Metabolism, nerves, and muscles
    Food sources: sunflower seeds, peas, pork, lima beans

8. Riboflavin: Formation of red blood cells, nervous system functions, and metabolism of carbs, protein, and fat
    Food sources: liver, whey, wheat germ, lamb, beef

9. Colalamin (Vitamin B12): Blood formation and nervous system health
    Food sources: oysters, lamb, beef, shellfish, poultry

10. Niacin: Metabolizes carbs, fat and protein; helps nervous system function
    Food sources: soy protein, whey protein, peanuts, sunflower seeds

11. Folic Acid: Growth, development and red blood cell formation; may decrease birth defects
    Food sources: brewer's yeast, beans, turnips, seaweed, eggs

12. Biotin: Assists in metabolism of fat and utilizes vitamin B
    Food sources: beef, liver, oyster, pork, fish, poultry

13. Pantothenic Acid: Aids growth and development
    Food sources: sunflower seeds, whey protein, soy, peanuts, broccoli, liver

Minerals

Needed for a variety of functions, including bone health, oxygen-carrying capacity, and the fluid and electrolyte balance.

1. Calcium: Develops and maintains bones and teeth; assists in blood clotting, muscle contraction, transmission of nerve impulses, and prevention of osteoporosis
   Food sources: fruit juice, cheese, milk, yogurt, cottage cheese, ice cream, kale, Chinese cabbage.

2. Phosphorus: Works with calcium for bone growth; essential for energy metabolism, DNA structure and cell membranes.
   Food sources: cheese, fish, whole wheat, cocoa powder, pumpkin seeds, almonds.

3. Magnesium: Helps nerve and muscle functions, constitution of bone and teeth
   Food sources: soy beans, nuts, spinach, brown rice

4. Molybdenum: Needed for metabolism of DNA and RNA, production of uric acid
   Food sources: liver, beans, peas

5. Manganese: Aids in metabolism of carbs; develops skeletal and connective tissue
   Food sources: wheat germ, whole wheat, wheat bran

6. Copper: Iron metabolism, nervous system function and bone health, protein synthesis, pigmentation of skin
   Food sources: liver, shellfish, lobster, nuts

7. Chromium: Aids in glucose metabolism, regulates blood sugar and insulin
   Food sources: raw oyster, wine, apple, pork

8. Iodine: Part of thyroid hormone, regulates growth, development, energy metabolism
   Food sources: iodized salt, sea food

9. Iron: Important for red blood cell formation and function
   Food sources: liver, beets, veal, kidney beans, almonds, cashew nuts

10. Selenium: Essential antioxidant, normal growth and development
    Food sources: tenderloin beef, trout, tuna, oysters, sunflower seeds, wheat germ, crab, cod

11. Zinc: Essential part of enzymes involved in digestion, metabolism, reproduction, wound healing
    Food sources: oyster, veal, lamb, chicken, peas, lima beans

Want Food
These foods can be harmful to your health.

PROCESSED, REFINED, AND INORGANIC FOOD

This is the type of food you often see at supermarkets. Want foods are easy, convenient foods; they are enjoyed by many, but they are addictive.

Processed food has little or no nutritive value (often labeled microwavable or quick fix and wrapped in plastic). It is loaded with chemicals, preservatives, colors, acids, and bleached to change the original nature of the food and increase shelf life.

Refined foods lack natural nutrients and fiber and offer a sweeter version of the original food. For example, fast food loaded with preservatives and additives to increase shelf life.

Compared with organic foods or inorganic whole foods, the chemicals in processed food enter your body and damage your cells and organs, and it's highly toxic. If it's inorganic food, it's safe to boil or grill before you eat it instead of eating it raw. Either option is lot better than eating refined or processed food.

When you see ingredients that are confusing and inaccurate, it's a red flag. Over the years, medical studies have shown that additives, colors, thickeners, emulsifiers, flavors, and preservatives are linked with certain types of cancers, stress, heart disease, diabetes, allergies, kidney and liver damage.

How to Select Food
Now we will look at how you can select food by reading the labels and before you choose whether to take it home or to put it back on the shelf.

FOUR REASONS TO PUT SOMETHING BACK ON THE SHELF

1) **Preservatives**
Most commonly used ingredients to increase shelf life: BHA (320), BHT (E321), nitrates (nitrites, sodium nitrate E250-251, E249252–Potassium nitrate; e.g., hot dogs, bacon and ham), nitrosamine, and monosodium glutamate MSG/621.

Flavor enhancers (can cause allergic reaction), monopotassium glutamate (622), Disodium Inosinate (631), benzoic acid, benzotates (E210–219). Examples: soda or beer.

2) **Emulsifiers, Stabilizers, and Thickener**
Found in sauces, soups, bread, cake, ice cream, chocolate and milk shakes.

Also, look out for sugar alternatives (sucrose, fructose, dextrose, corn syrup, maltodextrin).

Animal fat is saturated fat. Trans fat is hydrogenated fat.

Carcinogenic sweeteners: mannitol, sorbitol, xylitol, saccharine

Other chemicals which has a negative impact which are found in foods: ammonium, bicarbonate, malic acid, fumeric acid, lactic acid, lecithin, xanthan gum, calcium chloride, monocalcium phosphate, monopotassium sulphate.

3) **Coloring**
These could damage your immune system and speed aging.

Green, Blue, and Yellow: Tartrazine (E102), Quinolic Yellow (E104), Sunset Yellow (E110), Beetroot Red & Red (E162), Caramel (E150).

4) **Sweetners**
These are meant to enhance the natural sweetness in food thereby forming an addictive behavior for sweets and ultimately having a price tag linked with cancer.

Eg: E950 Pottasium Acesulphame, E951 Aspartame, E954 Saccharin

THREE REASONS TO TAKE FOOD HOME

1) If it's organic or inorganic whole, natural food.
2) If you can read or pronounce all the ingredients.
3) If it has a short expiration date with no added preservatives, coloring, or additives. For example: fruits, vegetables, fresh seafood, poultry, meats, nuts, seeds, and dairy.

The above information is intended as a guideline for making smarter choices when selecting food. Whenever possible, go for organic or inorganic whole and natural foods. If you don't have a choice, it's better to have frozen or canned fruits, vegetables, and fish instead of processed or fast foods, which often have added chemicals or use genetically modified products.

SECTION 10 — IMPORTANCE OF RECOVERY AND REST

Think of your body like your mobile device: It needs to be recharged with use.

Your body and mind both need to be recharged. This is called recovery, and it enables you to give 100% in your next training session or at work.

You could be drained of energy due to one or many of the reasons mentioned below:

1. Energy drain: during repetitive demands, decrease in nutrition, or decrease in hydration

2. Muscle drain: from high-intensity exercises

3. Mental drain: from injury or lack of motivation

4. Emotional drain: This is psychological and mainly outside of training (problems or stress from family, school, work, and relationships). This should be addressed by a qualified professional.

5. Environmental fatigue: climate change, deviating from your wake-up time, bedtime, meals etc.

Since we already discussed the importance of nutrition in the previous section, we can proceed to look at the other factors.

Sleep
This is the best type of recovery. Getting seven to nine hours of sleep is a must for physical, emotional, neurological, and immunological stress relief. Kids might need around ten hours of sleep.

If you sleep more than this, it slows the central nervous system by producing melatonin (hormone associated with your sleeping and waking up cycles), which leads to lethargy.

Napping more than ten minutes will upset your sleep quality as well.

Lack of sleep can cause the following problems.
1) Irritability
2) Increased heart rate
3) Increased risk of heart disease
4) Improper judgment
5) Decreased Immunity
6) Decreased growth
7) Increased reaction time
8) Decreased accuracy
9) Tremors

To be in line with the scope of this book, taking one or two rest days per week is recommended. During this period, do not engage in much physical activity. Instead, you could socialize, shop, or play with your pet (if applicable).

Unless you are in a supervised conditioning program for a specific sport, do not get into the habit of playing the same sport throughout the year, as this will lead to repetitive stress and could cause injury.

Kids should be allowed to play multiple sports to develop their overall athletic abilities (e.g., tennis, basketball, soccer, and swimming).

Each sport has its own dominant activity pattern and energy patterns, so children will develop athletic abilities. They can specialize when they grow into teenagers and find a proper sports coach and a conditioning coach.

Adults should select a sport as a recreational activity. Apart from your gym visits and using the treadmill, bicycles, aerobic classes, and other group classes, most adults have the goals of weight loss and being healthy and injury-free in performing daily tasks. You may choose hiking, Pilates, Tennis BPM, surfing, scuba diving, Latin dancing, yoga, squash, basketball, or swimming.

The variety of following these guidelines will provide you with physical benefits that you wouldn't get participating in a single sport all year.

Relaxation

Individuals respond differently to stressful situations such as anger, anxiety, and tiredness. Here are some ways you can practice relaxation.

1) **Hydrotherapy**
   This is one of the most famous methods of relaxation. From ancient times up to the current sports world, it's an integral part of training.
   a) Pools (light active movement)
   b) Steam rooms/ice baths will provide hot and cold temperatures to increase or reduce blood flow.

2) **Massage, Self-Massage, Foam Rollers**
   Targets superficial and deep muscles, connective tissues, and skin; increases blood flow by applying pressure, tension, motion and vibration.
   Positive effects: Pain relief; decreases anxiety, depression, blood pressure, and heart rate. It also stimulates endorphins associated with pain killers and the feel-good hormone serotonin associated with excitement, pain, and love.

Some other common relaxation methods are mentioned below.

1) **Autogenic Training**
   Daily participation of 10–15 minutes, 2–3 times a day; visualizing something pleasant and repeating it makes an individual relax.
   Examples: Tropical island with a waterfall or listening to the sound of birds.

2) **Deep Breathing**
   Called abdominal breathing; not chest breathing. This will introduce more oxygen into the system.
   Close your eyes and keep your palms on your stomach; breathe in for 10–15 counts, and then breathe out for 10–15 counts.

3) **Meditation**
   This is self-consciousness; it's an internal practice.
   It calms the parasympathetic nervous system via reduction of noise and stimulation.
   This practice can control blood pressure, decrease an elevated heart rate, slow breathing rhythms, relax muscles, and calm the sympathetic nervous system (when you are overstimulated).

4) Progressive Muscle Relaxation (PMR)

Can reduce anxiety, insomnia and hypertension

1. Sit or lie down with your eyes closed.
2. Visualize your body, feet to head or vice versa.
3. Contract each muscle for 10 seconds and relax for 20 seconds.
4. Through awareness and practice, you can relax your tight muscles.

5) Visualization

This is a popular method among professional athletes to generate game scenarios; imagine real-situations or a relaxing vacation that made your mind and body calm.

This method uses senses to create the image (sound, touch, smell, and sight) for reality-based visualizations.

For example: Visualize swimming in a beach area. Feel the waves, salty water, breeze, and sunshine.

6) Music

Can be used to motivate or relax, depending on individual tastes. Try the suggested categories below as you select your own music.

a) Wake up: Disco
b) While at work: Lounge
c) Working out: Rock
d) Stressed out: Instrumental
e) Motivation: Music that inspires you (of any genre)
f) Sleeping: Nature sounds

SAMPLE PROGRAMS FOR KIDS, TEENS, AND ADULTS

This section provides a basic description of how to set up a program for different age groups to suit their individual goals. Your certified trainer will guide you towards attaining your specific goals.

1) **Stability, Agility and Coordination Program for Kids**

   Warm-up
   - Exercises 1–10 (Section 1, p. 12–16): 8–10 min.

   Stability (Section 3) 8–10 min.
   - Lower-body stability with both feet (p. 22): 10 sec., 4 sets
   - Single-leg stability (p. 23): 10 reps, 3 sets
   - Upper-body stability (p. 24): 10 sec., 3 sets
   - Alternative dynamic stability (p. 23): 2 sets

   Coordination (Section 4): 4 sets, 10 min.
   - Foot-eye coordination (p. 29)
   - Hand-eye coordination (p. 29)

   Agility (Section 6): 4–6 sets
   - Cone T drill (p. 73)
   - Ladder crossover step (p. 78)

   Flexibility (Section 8)
   - Exercises 1–9 and 11, 13, 14 (p. 86–93)

2) **Muscle Conditioning Program for Teens**

Warm-up (Section 1, p. 12–16)
- Exercises: 1, 2, 3, 4, 8, 9

Basic conditioning (Section 5)
- Dumbbell squat (p. 37)
- Dumbbell press (p. 46)
- Dumbbell lunge (p. 37)
- Dumbbell close pull (p. 52)
- Dumbbell side press (p. 60)
- Dumbbell calves (p. 40)
- Dumbbell hammer curls (p. 55)
- Dumbbell triceps extension (p. 56)
- Ab crunch (p. 64)
- Ab rotation (p. 63)
- Floor quad lift (p. 68)

Cooldown and flexibility (Section 8)
- Exercises 1–17 (p. 86–95)

3) **Calorie Burning Workout for Adults**

Warm-up (Section 1, p. 12–16): 8–10 min.

Stability (Section 3)
- Single-leg stability (p. 23): 10 reps, 2 sets on each leg
- Upper-body alternate-arm stability (p. 24): 10 reps, 3–4 sets
- Core stability (p. 25): 20 sec., 4–5 sets

Muscle conditioning (Section 5)
- Band squat (p. 35)
- Band chest rotation (p. 44)
- Band rotation backward (p. 49)
- Band shoulder press (p. 58)
- Band crunches (p. 63)
- Band back reach (p. 67)

Agility (Section 6)
- Cone T drill (p. 73)
- Ladder side shuffle (p. 77)

Reaction and quickness (Section 7)
- Reaction ball catch and bounce (p. 79)
- Copy partner (p. 81)

Cardiovascular and respiratory (Section 2)
- CV with basketball, medicine ball, or tennis ball (p. 19)

Cooldown and flexibility (Section 8)
- Exercises 1–17 (p. 86–95)

FINAL NOTE

I hope you have a new understanding of how important exercise, nutrition, rest, and recovery are. I have tried to make this book easy to read by omitting technical and scientific words as much as possible and by keeping the content to a minimum. I'm a firm believer that one can learn from books, but if you don't apply that knowledge to your daily life, it's a waste of time.

My clients and athletes are motivated because I practice what I preach. Similarly, you should do what you read as long it's sensible and supported with valid reason.

Visit www.TennisBPM.com for more sample programs, video clips, and articles on health and fitness.

You may also visit the website to find out more about workshops and seminars on how to train pro athletes on different components of fitness or to get certified in Tennis BPM.

WARNING

Please consult your physician (primary care practitioner) before participation in the exercises or following the nutrition guidelines described in this book or participating in any other physical activity or nutritional strategies. This book is for informational purposes only. The author and publisher are not liable for any injury or health risks associated with participating in the exercise or nutritional strategies described in this book. It is advisable that you always work with accredited fitness professionals after gaining the approval of your physician.

BIBLIOGRAPHY

1. Elliot, B., Reid, M., and Crespo, M. (2003). *Biomechanics of Advanced Tennis.* London: ITF.

2. Chu, D. (1998). *Jumping into Plyometrics.* Champaign, IL: Human Kinetics.

3. Reid, M., Quinn, A., and Crespo, M. (2003). *Strength and Conditioning for Tennis.* London: ITF.

4. William, S. (2000). *Serious Tennis.* Champaign, IL: Human Kinetics.

5. Chu, D. (1995). *Power Tennis Training.* Champaign, IL: Human Kinetics.

6. Foran, B. (2001). *High Performance Sports Conditioning.* Champaign, IL: Human Kinetics.

7. Murphy, S. (2005). *The Sport Psych Handbook.* Champaign, IL: Human Kinetics.

8. Griffith, W. and Friscia, D. (2004). *The Complete Guide to Sports Injuries.* New York: Penguin Group.

9. Pluim, B. and Safran, M. (2004). *From Breakpoint to Advantage.* Vista, CA: Racquet Tech Publishing.

10. ACSM (2007). *Guidelines for Exercise Testing and Prescription.* Baltimore: William and Wilkins.

11. Bompa, T. (2000). *Total Training for Young Champions.* Peoria, IL: Versa Press.

12.   Beachle, T. and Earle, R. (2000) *NSCA: Essentials of Strength Training and Conditioning*. Champaign, IL: Human Kinetics.

13.   Clark, M. and Lucett, S. (2010). *NASM: Essentials of Sports Performance Training*. Baltimore: William and Wilkins.

14.   Garrison, R. and Sommers, E. (1995). *Nutrition Desk Reference*. New Canaan, CT: Keats Publishing, Inc.

15.   Houtkooper, L., Abbot, J. and Mullis, V. (2007). *Winning Sports Nutrition*. AZ: Desert Southwest Fitness, Inc.

16.   Bompa, T. (1994). *Periodization: Training for Sports*. Peoria, IL: Versa Press.

17.   Morgan, G.T. and Mcglynn, G.H (1997). *Cross-Training for Sports*. Peoria, IL: Versa Press.

18.   Mcginnis, P. (1999). *Biomechanics of Sports and Exercise*. Champaign, IL: Human Kinetics.

19.   Fleck, S.J. and Kramer, W.J. (1997). *Designing Resistance Training Programs*, 2nd ed. Champaign, IL: Human Kinetics.

20.   Costello, F. and Kresis, E.J. (1993). *Sports Agility*. Nashville, TN: Taylor Sports.

21.   Hatfield, F.C. (1989). *Power: A Scientific Approach*. Chicago: Contemporary Books, Inc.

22.   USTA (1998). *Complete Conditioning for Tennis*. Champaign, IL: Human Kinetics.

23.   Grosser, M., Kraft, H., and Schonborn, R. (2000). *Speed Training for Tennis*. Oxford: Myer and Meyer Sports (UK), Ltd.

24.   Durbik, J. (1996). Children and Sports Training. Island Pond, VT: Stadion Publishing Co.

25.   Nye, A. (2004). *First Aid Handbook*. Bath: Parragon Publishing.

26.   "Overview of Food Ingredients, Additives and Colors," U.S. Food and Drug Administration website. http://www.fda.gov/Food/IngredientsPackagingLabeling/ FoodAdditivesIngredients/ucm094211.htm.

27.   "Complete Lists of Additives," Food Intolerance Network, http://fedup.com.au/ information/information/complete-lists-of-additives-3.

28.   "Additives and Preservatives," Faqs.org. http://www.faqs.org/nutrition/A-Ap/ Additives-and-Preservatives.html.

www.ingramcontent.com/pod-product-compliance
Lightning Source LLC
Chambersburg PA
CBHW080955290526
45795CB00009B/2957